the **TRUTH** ABOUT **BEAUTY**

the TRUTH ABOUT BEAUTY

BEAUTY

TRANSFORM YOUR LOOKS AND YOUR LIFE FROM THE INSIDE OUT

KAT JAMES

BEYOND
WORDS
Publishing

Beyond Words Publishing, Inc.
20827 N.W. Cornell Road, Suite 500
Hillsboro, Oregon 97124-9808
503-531-8700

The author and the publisher gratefully acknowledge and thank the following for permission to reprint previously published material quoted in this book:

Excerpts from "The Makeup-less Makeover," by Kat James, edited by Jerry Shaver, *Better Nutrition*, October 2002. Copyright © 2002 by Sabot Publishing, Inc. Reprinted by permission of *Better Nutrition*.

Excerpts from "Things to Do to Honor Your True Beauty," from the Web site of The IDentity Project.® Reprinted by permission of Communicating the Power of One, Inc.

Editors: Jenefer Angell and Julie Steigerwaldt
Copy editor: Jade Chan
Proofreader: Marvin Moore
Design: Angela Lavespere
Composition: William H. Brunson Typography Services

Printed in the United States of America
Distributed to the book trade by Publishers Group West

Library of Congress Cataloging-in-Publication Data
James, Kat.
    The truth about beauty : transform your looks and your life from the inside out / Kat James.
       p. cm.
    Includes bibliographical references and index.
    ISBN 1-58270-100-8
    1. Beauty, Personal.   2. Women—Health and hygiene.   3. Holistic medicine. I. Title.

RA778.J274   2003
646.7′042—dc21

                  2003009861

The corporate mission of Beyond Words Publishing, Inc.:
Inspire to Integrity

dedication

To the woman I was—for whom this book would have been a godsend—and to all women and men who seek to regain radiance and mastery over their own physical destinies

In memory of Allyn Farmer

contents

PART III: THE MAKEUP-LESS MAKEOVER

disclaimer

Dear Reader:

Please understand that the information, scientific studies, specific solutions, and opinions discussed in this book, while carefully researched, are offered for educational purposes only. They are not intended as diagnoses or treatments for specific ailments or replacements for the expertise of your qualified healthcare provider. If you feel that certain information applies to a health-related issue of your own, it is crucial that you bring it to the attention of your healthcare provider for confirmation and treatment. The use of any of this information without consulting a physician may be dangerous. Neither the publisher nor the author accepts responsibility for any effects that may arise from the correct or incorrect use of information in this book.

My goal is to awaken your excitement, skepticism, curiosity, and hunger for more information so that you may grab the reins and direct your own path to your true, vital health and beauty potential.

Legal notice: The health-related statements in this book have not been evaluated by the U.S. Food and Drug Administration.

foreword

The Truth about Beauty presents a timely and powerful departure from standard health and diet practices. I find that too many beauty and health experts—including some of my colleagues in the nutrition field—are disconnected with what really make or breaks people's ability to look their best and treat themselves in the most caring and healthful way. Kat James not only uncovers these missing pieces, she gives us the physical tools to look and live better than ever—no matter where we start from.

Kat and I share a connection because we both bring a personal story of transformation to our work. Kat sees the potential in everyday people that most cannot envision for themselves. This book will help readers uncover that physical potential and avoid the extreme, tedious—even dangerous—measures we've been programmed to believe are necessary. Anyone who takes an interest in his or her health and beauty will find powerful inspiration in these pages, in addition to well honed, practical tips that yield marked improvements in lifestyle.

Because Kat is not a beauty or diet "spokesmodel" or a product of fantastic genes, a Hollywood upbringing, or personal trainers and chefs, she represents the real possibility for any woman to transform herself without obsession and without committing herself to drastic skin or diet regimens or a commando's workout program. Kat understands all of the points of resistance: what it's like to lack motivation, to prefer certain tastes, to be skeptical or leery of suggestions that are unappealing or ineffective, or simply to live in a geographical location without easy access to good food and products. Kat deftly navigates all of these and turns them all in the reader's favor.

Kat James's approach challenges several basic notions that many in my field rely on when they run out of answers. She provides a much-needed wake-up call for the millions of people who could benefit from her message. In addition, I strongly recommend Kat's teachings to therapists, doctors, fitness trainers, and other nutritionists looking to increase their insights into health, beauty, and wellness and to improve success with their clients. With *The Truth about Beauty*, Kat James raises the bar for other books in the field by closing the chapter on outmoded, standard diet and skin advice and opening a new way of achieving the beauty that is everyone's birthright.

Oz Garcia

acknowledgments

There are many people without whom this book would not have been "born" and to whom I wish to extend my deepest gratitude:

To Michael Broussard, for believing in and selling something so impossible to explain! To Julie Steigerwaldt, my managing editor, for guiding and delivering my "baby" true to form. To Jenefer Angell, for helping me shape it. To Cynthia Black and Richard Cohn at Beyond Words, as well as Jan Miller, for letting me do the book I was born to do. And to Marvin Moore, Jade Chan, Angela Lavespere, Bill Brunson, Sylvia Hayse, Beth Hoyt, and Dorral Lukas, as well as Holly Taylor, for their hours of work and expertise.

A very special thanks to the amazing Oz Garcia, B.S., M.A., for writing the foreword. To Dr. Nicholas Perricone, Dr. Susan Lark, Dr. Michael B. Schachter, Dr. David Edelson, and Dr. Deborah Jaliman, for their compelling interviews and pioneering insights. To Lauren Rogers of the IDentity Project and Communicating the Power of One, for contributing the list "Things to Do to Honor Your True Beauty" in Part I. And to John Monahan, Danny Vincent, Patrycja Towns, and Jerry Shaver at *Better Nutrition* magazine, for giving me incredible support and a voice through such a great magazine and for use of Jerry's deft edit of my personal story for Part I of this book.

Many thanks to the pioneering authors, researchers, and journalists whose work has helped shape my overall perspective and has contributed to this book, including Dr. Barry Sears, Dr. Samuel S. Epstein, Annemarie Colbin, Dr. Julian Whitaker, Dr. Stephen Cherniske, Dr. Rudy Rivera, Burton Goldberg, Dr. Aubrey Hampton, Dr. James A. Duke, Michael T. Murray, N.D., Dr. Alan Gaby, Udo Erasmus, Dr. Russell L. Blaylock, Nicolas J. Smeh, M.S., Ruth Winter, Kim Erikson, Judi Vance, Lindsey Berkson, Michael Pollan, Gary Taubes, and the Life Extension Foundation, as well as the many researchers who've spent countless hours in labs contributing to the published science that supports this book. And to the late Dr. Robert Atkins, without whom the conventional American dietary paradigm might still be frozen in time.

To the women whose stories I share in this book.

To Stephen Churchill Downes, for the very special cover photo. And to Barry Yee, for shooting the author photo.

To the following individuals who have gone out of their way to mentor or support my journey to publishing: Jim Indorato, Maureen O'Brien, Jory Des Jardin, Kate White, Andrea Clark, Mary Rose Almasi, Janet Parker, Neal Hirschfeld, Suzanne Grimes, Jill White, Liz Smith, Ryan Kuhn, Bruce Marcus, Bev Matson, Pratima Raichur, N.D., Susan Hussey, Stephanie Von Hirshberg, Roger Itkor, Lois Johnson, Annika Hayes, Ailsa Long, Alexis Luce of Luce Consulting, Doug Bolin, Lyle Hurd, Jerry Isley, John and Kristin Armstrong, Lois Greenfield, Jennifer Greenwald, Linda Roemer, Tori Rowan, Cameron Wolbert, Lawrence Rosen, Kristina Sachs, Dennis Tarr, Nancy Trent at Trent and Company, Linda Bryer at Bryer Advertising and Public Relations, Caroline MacDougall, Jane Iredale, Cheryl Roth and Mara Engel at OrganicWorks Marketing, Marilyn Dale, Cindy Connelly, Wanda Daniels, Walter Seigordner, Kim Sayer, Karin Miksche, Mary Cooper, and Kristen Knowles.

To my mother, Suzanne Farmer, for encouraging every road I've taken and for giving me her writing "genes." To Jon and Julie Farmer, for their encouragement and review of material. To Tom and Dave and their families, for their lovingness throughout the duration of my prolonged solitude. To Lance Rieck, Joseph Bongiourno, Bruce Crossland, Scott Allerding, Cynthia Faye, and especially Robert Morningstar, for watching over me. And finally to Peter Verlander, Ph.D., for endless research help, for playing the ultimate devil's advocate, for showing me my strength, and without whose material support and companionship this book would not have been possible.

introduction

our beauty needs a sanctuary

Have you ever been captivated by someone whose beauty seemed to transcend sex, sex appeal, and age? Why were you so riveted? Was it confidence? Grace? When that person moved closer, the classic features you had expected to see did not appear. Instead, despite facial flaws and asymmetries, you saw what had captivated you more clearly: a glow. Sparkling eyes and vibrant skin delicately etched with the signs of a rich and expressive life projected a sense of calm and a focused demeanor. Suddenly you knew you were beholding the most precious and elusive beauty attribute of all: vitality.

Untold vitality lies within each of us. To connect with it, we must build a sanctuary far from the constant physical and sensory bombardments and life challenges that can take a toll on our inner and outer beauty. In that sacred space, we can rise above the fray, retrace our steps, face eye-opening facts, and reprogram the mind-sets that led us to the choices that have kept us from our vital essence. Armed with solid motivation, empowering and accurate information, and the wisest lifestyle choices, we discover that true radiance and beauty is readily accessible when we uncover and re-hone our beauty instincts. With renewed confidence, we can safely and deftly navigate the modern beauty labyrinth.

My motivation for writing this book runs deep. As a teenager, I developed a compulsive eating disorder that dominated my life for twelve years. That bleak period included the first five years of my career as a makeup artist in New York City, where I worked with celebrities such as Sarah Jessica Parker and Martha Stewart and would eventually act as a spokesperson for cosmetic brands such as Maybelline and Revlon and enjoy the spotlight as a TV makeover guru. But despite my deftness at making others beautiful on the outside, it wasn't until I was twenty-six that a physical crisis forced me to face my own biggest beauty challenge: to win the compulsive battle against my body and my self that deprived me of my self-respect, my looks, and eventually my health. It took this life-altering event for me to transcend the hair and makeup cover-ups I had depended on for so long and change everything I thought I knew about beauty.

Ironically, my real beauty story began when I finally let go of my superficial beauty goals. Motivated in an entirely new way, I stumbled upon a better world of information and options that not only freed me from my eating disorder but from the self-sabotage, broken diets, and physical complaints that came with it. Shedding ten dress sizes was the most physically obvious sign of my breakthrough, but it was a mere side effect of a greater victory: getting my life back and discovering my real beauty potential for the first time.

Today the woman I am is unrecognizable from the woman I was. The path from the depleted, disconnected life I once lived to the way I live and look today had nothing to do with hard work, sweat, or deprivation. My escape from the physical fate nature had never intended for me resulted from a complete reprogramming of my concepts of beauty, how to get a great body, and how to live life to the fullest.

In the years since my transformation, I have worked with dozens of women and touched thousands more via my Web site, magazine columns, workshops, and other avenues. These women seek a more authentic path to physical radiance and an escape from the modern merry-go-round of problem-causing self-care regimens. With the help of the strategies and information in this book, many of them have been able to change not only their reflections in the mirror but also their lives. In the pages that follow, I will share stories drawn from their ongoing transformations.

My formal training is in aesthetics and cosmetology, not healthcare. I'm not a doctor, nutritionist, or dermatologist, and this book is not intended as a prescription or treatment but as a source of information. I encourage healthy skepticism, and I present the scientific research to validate each area of my approach. I hope to help you as I have helped others: by inspiring you with my own transformation and giving you the incentive and tools with which to take control of your own life.

my promise: vitality has untold plans for each of us

The Truth about Beauty is designed to lift the spirit and tap into the unique vital essence in all of us. It is not about striving for a beauty ideal dictated by our culture. Our impulse is to impose our own visions and ideals on our physical selves; however, we have the ability to create something and someone even more stunning—if we get out of its way and allow it to emerge. We were all meant to be beautiful. Even those without the problem that I had can expect the return of something they thought was youth—which was really just health—and the emergence of something—or some*one*— they've never seen before.

My goal is to guide you and introduce you to the tools that you can use today to begin your transformation. As you become increasingly conscious of the inseparable connection between health and beauty, you'll soon find that once the process has started, it begins to perpetuate and inspire itself.

As you go from one amazing reward to the next, your beauty, your sensibilities, and your quality of life will evolve, often to unprecedented levels, and allow an ageless radiance to emerge.

In part I, "Uncovering Your True Radiant Potential," I'll share my journey from being a compulsive, denatured woman to the health crisis that led me to a world of information and the invaluable tools that helped me heal my body, uncover my beauty, and free myself from my battles with willpower and self-sabotage forever. To establish your own starting point, you'll take a dawn-to-dusk self-inventory.

In part II, "Feeding and Cultivating Beauty," I'll encourage you to become a "food snob" by providing you with science-backed beauty incentives. I'll introduce you to a series of food and beverage upgrades that take you from beauty-robbing choices to body-decadent pleasures. I'll then clarify the factors in food addiction and how to starve its support system without starving yourself. You'll then discover how supplements can transform not only your relationship with food but also your looks and your life.

In part III, "The Makeup-less Makeover," you'll learn how to recover your skin's own self-rejuvenating functions and gain a broader perspective of the proven ways to resolve stubborn skin issues. You'll gain an understanding of how to minimize the beauty "wild cards" that jeopardize your most radiant potential. And finally, I'll show you how to let your beauty ripple outward with the choices you make every day.

I don't believe in disrupting routines or giving up convenience in order to live well and stay beautiful, which is why I wouldn't dream of writing this book without also including a listing of products and services to help you simply and joyfully upgrade your lifestyle. As you learn how to evaluate what goes on and in your body in an informed way, you can use the "Living Beauty Resource Guide" as a key source to help you satisfy your evolving criterion.

Though I freely give my opinions, I don't want to dictate another list of rules for you to blindly follow. Instead, I want to empower you to make your own informed choices based on the whole picture. By painlessly upgrading each area of your life, you can experience stunning short- and long-term rewards such as a re-emergence of your healthiest glow (without blush or foundation), revitalized skin (without harsh regimens), the end of dry skin (without heavy lotions), diminished under-eye circles, shrunken varicose veins, glossier hair, youthful energy, freedom from cravings, and—best of all—an energetic, comfortable new body that adjusts to your ideal weight, without drugs, diets, or formal workouts. Your taste buds will become more discerning, and you will relish your meals. You will be happier about the way you look and feel, and you will find that these lifestyle changes are not only rewarding to your body and spirit but can be effortlessly and joyfully maintained forever.

Many readers will be surprised at how easy some of the most powerfully transforming lifestyle adjustments can be and how quickly the benefits can be seen and felt. Beauty never forgets its essence, even if we—and our world—have. Given any opportunity, beauty will reestablish itself. My tools for transformation can be used by people of any age, size, or shape—and, yes, gender. In fact, the more challenged you are at the start, the more dramatic your rewards will be. Think about where I started. Think where you could go.

I invite you to begin your journey of self-discovery with these strategies and from there to experiment, question, and take pleasure in tailoring your new self-care habits to help create the most fulfilling life possible. Real sanctuary from toxic and sensory bombardment includes a break from the countless assaults hidden in our personal care and beauty regimens. With each layer of beauty baggage that you shed, your perspective will also evolve as you look back in amazement on the way you used to care for yourself. You will rejoice to be free of your misconceptions as a whole new world of possibilities and a whole new level of connection with your intended radiance and your *self* opens up.

Part 1

UNCOVERING YOUR TRUE RADIANT POTENTIAL

the **ULTIMATE BEAUTY LESSON**

I was twenty-four, living in New York City, and lying in bed after my usual binge—this time it was each flavor of Rosa's fudge from the deli across the street. When I could eat no more, my heart started pounding. I was scared, but I forced myself to lie still. I tried to breathe deeply and make my heart calm down, but the pounding wouldn't stop. "What makes you do this?" I thought. "What are you afraid of?" I opened my diary as I so often did after a binge. I would write passages from self-help books or tally my calorie intake, and in the spirit of creative accounting, I would carry the "spill over" to the next day's allotment. I was addicted to starting over. But at this point I was beyond writing about the old emotional triggers, tallying all the calories I'd just consumed, or planning a new diet to try tomorrow. None of those plans had ever worked.

I flipped back through the pages of my journal, through all my accumulated lists of when-I-get-thin dreams—the dancer, the singer, the Broadway performer, the person who would get back at those who had rejected her. There were so many things I had planned to do when I got thin.

Then I suddenly imagined doing *none* of them and letting myself off the hook. In my journal, I gave myself permission to fail, to not even attempt to reach these goals. I promised myself the kind of padding from the world that my weight problem and my unhealthy relationship with food had always given me—both literally and figuratively. I could remain antisocial, give up perfectionism, let go of those when-I-get-thin dreams, and love myself anyway. It was such a wild concept; I took it to heart for the first time in my life.

It was a radical stretch for a perfectionist, but I made myself believe it as I pledged to stop judging myself harshly and to let go of the demands on the person I'd be if I were thin. "It's OK to fail!" I wrote. Suddenly I felt the kind of relief you felt as a kid on a snow day when you learned that there was no school and nothing was expected of you. I fell asleep with the peace you feel after a good cry. I had no idea that the next morning would be different from the ones before or that I had just solved the final piece of a multi-faceted puzzle that I had struggled with for twelve years.

In the morning I was surprised to feel that same sense of peace. When I looked in the mirror, instead of the shame and self-loathing my reflection normally evoked, I saw my body for the first time as an "innocent," lovable creation that had been distorted by years of abuse. It was as if I'd become my own ideal mother seeing her battered child at the front door after a terrible journey. I had never felt such an outpouring of love and sadness from my heart to my body as I did then. That feeling of peace stayed with me as that day turned into weeks. I have never binged again and have never even been compelled to.

early signs

When I was thirteen, I started a string of diets. It was during these first attempts at calorie restriction that I began to binge. By high school, I was a fan of tunics and wore a thick mask of painstakingly applied makeup to distract from my conspicuously pear-shaped body. I'd been a singer and dancer since childhood, but my talent couldn't land me the roles or scholarships I wanted—until my senior year, when I discovered speed pills and began purging. I lost more than twenty pounds. I got the lead in the school play, the boyfriend, the choir scholarship, the dance solo. It was like a dream—until the school cracked down on the supplier of my magic pills. It wasn't easy to watch the weight pile back on. The taste of glory I'd had made the years that followed all the more painful.

In college my weight yo-yoed between 140 and 185 pounds. By the time I was twenty, I'd become a physically distorted beauty statistic of our times—heavy, but well coiffed, meticulously made up, manicured, perfumed, powdered, and groomed, yet riddled with uncomfortable skin rashes, digestive troubles, allergies, and an unbelievably powerful addiction to food.

At that time I began to look for books that addressed the emotional causes for my self-destructive behavior. I collected resounding pieces of wisdom from various self-help books. I read about the healing power of self-expression, the destructive power of guilt, the inner child, the fact that feelings aren't debatable, and the risks and ultimate rewards of vulnerability. Perhaps the most important theory I learned was the self-defeating trap of indefinite blame. At the dawn of my twenties, I carried years and layers of heavy resentment toward my mother and had become emotionally paralyzed by the weight of that burden, waiting for apologies and becoming more and more resentful each day I didn't get them. In her, I'd found an eternal excuse not to fully address my eating problem myself. Then I finally realized that even if, by some miracle, I were to receive the apologies that I craved, I still would be stuck in a quagmire from which only I could free myself. I identified and addressed these emotional triggers, and I felt a great weight being lifted as I dropped that old baggage, but to my frustration, my physical compulsion to binge and my torturous daily battle with food remained strong. With no escape in sight, I gave up my performing-arts scholarship, dropped out of college, and enrolled in beauty school. I later joined my sister in New York City and became a makeup artist, since I'd always been good at making *others* look beautiful.

In late 1988 I arrived in New York City with looks that certainly attracted attention, thanks to the "stunning"—if not shocking—makeup and antigravity hair imported from Michigan and a backside that won the elusive New York City doubletake. For someone with my body and my background to pursue a career in beauty and fashion was a bit naïve, even masochistic. Everything about me was wrong for the world I was trying to penetrate. I didn't look like, dress, or act like any of the top makeup artists who worked with supermodels and celebrities. I wasn't skinny, artsy, or eccentric, and I didn't have an attitude. On the bright side, my sister's connections eventually led to an interview with Frederic Fekkai, one of the world's top celebrity hairdressers. When I think of what I wore to that interview—even the cab driver asked if I was "from around here"—I can't believe I was hired.

Working with models wasn't so bad. I regarded them as an elegant alien species. I felt no resentment toward them once I adjusted to my place in that world. Next to the models, I was like "Pat" from *Saturday Night Live*, a kind of asexual presence on the set. I suffered moments of extreme mortification, especially on location shoots when everyone was dying to jump into the ocean in their string bikinis after a hot day shooting on the beach and I was merely dying to escape the situation, get back to my hotel room, and binge yet again.

my first taste of real food

There were some unexpected upsides to big city living and working in fashion. The catered food on photo shoots was a revelation. Who knew that while I was growing up eating instant noodles and iceberg salads, other humans regularly dined on grainy pilafs, grilled vegetables, goat cheese, and herb-encrusted fish? I grew up in the fruit belt, which was really the Hamburger Helper and Shake 'n' Bake belt. I had never seen deep green lettuce or drunk mineral water (*without* ice) with meals. I soon learned that not all vegetables need to be cooked senseless and smothered beyond recognition in order to be edible. I'd always been leery of "health food," but these delicately cooked, aromatic dishes began to change my palate and my views. I began to judge a good salad based on new criteria, not because it was covered with Thousand Island dressing, croutons, and artificial bacon bits. Had I not moved to New York City, I may never have developed a taste for what I have come to call "real food."

I soon came to realize that eating this way all the time would be the ultimate luxury, though one I could not afford without giving up some of my other splurges. And so after giving up a few lipsticks and manicures, I was eating—and bingeing on—more real food. While changing my palate didn't change my need to use food as a drug, I was becoming a convert to quality vegetables and whole grains, yet I also ordered two or three desserts when I called for delivery. I continued to binge daily, both alone and on the job. I was good at sneaking several portions while other crew members socialized, and I *owned* the dessert tray, generously leaving one of each kind of pastry for the rest of the crew to nibble on. (That's what models do: nibble a *corner* off a brownie, which drove me crazy.) After days or weeks of bingeing, I would muster up epic willpower and eat nearly nothing or binge on low-calorie foods, such as frozen yogurt or soup, for a few days or sometimes even weeks. A handful of times I was able to starve myself down to near-normal size, functioning on loads of diet soda and frozen yogurt, thinking about food every waking moment.

I didn't have much of a social life. I much preferred the company of food to that of people. I would even leave friends' gatherings early to go home and eat. My journal writing continued to get me through the lows when my outlook was so bleak that I would occasionally stay in bed for days. Sometimes I would write down the reasons I had to live and remind myself of all the things I would do once I became thin. Then, of course, I would plan a new diet, set a new weight goal and deadline, and plan yet another drastic strategy.

Eventually, I decided to look into liposuction. The first two doctors I consulted refused to perform the procedure, saying it would be too dangerous unless I lost twenty pounds. The third doctor I saw agreed to do it and even offered a discount if he threw in a knee and abdomen suction. I started to save my money for the procedure, but I never went through with it.

a wake-up call

When I was twenty-four, my body began to break down. It started with fatigue and heart palpitations. The heart-pounding trudge up the subway stairs had become dreaded misery. Then came the blurry vision on mornings after a binge. But when I finally began passing undigested material (I was actually happy because I wasn't absorbing those calories), I decided to see a doctor. From a liver specialist I learned that I had a severely inflamed liver and prediabetic symptoms. I was looking at a lifetime of taking immuno-suppressants with notorious psychiatric and immune-system side effects.

This revelation jolted me into an entirely different perspective; in that moment I forgot about the scale, my diet, and the size 10 jeans I wanted to fit into. My decade-long preoccupation with weight completely vanished, and, for the first time, the "thin" dreams that had sustained me emotionally began to fade as my vision narrowed on my only beacon of hope: regaining my health.

However, this time I wasn't compelled to head to the gym or deprive myself of food. Rather, I started to read everything I could find about my liver condition and health in general. I bought my first non-diet health books at a health-food store, and they all mentioned the same herb in relation to my condition: milk thistle. Herbalists and alternative doctors seemed to agree about its value in healing the liver, which surprised me since I had always figured that herbology was the product of flowery imaginations. But I was willing to take the herbs and a leap of faith, in light of my grim prognosis. I needed to believe that I could thrive again. After seeing an alternative doctor who confirmed the benefits of milk thistle, I added other supplements to my regimen and took them religiously.

Two months later my liver enzymes were normal, down from the five-hundred range to a normal thirty-five. The liver specialist asked me what I had done. As I began to tell him, his eyes glazed over and he stopped listening to me. Like him, I had thought the treatment might have been a fluke. But after its success, I was irreversibly intrigued by alternative medicine and began reading more books about the other health problems and symptoms I had.

Up until then, I could not have imagined being interested in a book without an ideal weight or calorie chart that didn't specifically address weight loss. But these new books were different from typical nutrition and diet books. They skipped the typical talk about food pyramids, calorie limits, and fat grams. Instead, they focused on how different foods act in the body and even on what happens when we don't eat certain kinds of foods (and fats) or get certain nutrients over a long period of time. Until I read these books, I had never imagined that I could possibly have been deprived of *anything*, since I was always recovering from having eaten too much. And any periods of "successful" deprivation and great willpower—going for weeks eating only frozen yogurt, soup, and rice cakes and sipping diet soda—were what I had equated with victory and being "good."

My food research led me to begin reading about body-care products, which as a beauty professional, I had never considered from a health standpoint—other than to avoid blinding a client. I was shocked to learn how we absorb and accumulate many of these substances, and I became determined to eliminate as many internal and external irritants as I could from my life. I wanted to *thrive*, not just *react*, to my choices. And I knew that this is what my body—with all its health and skin discomforts—had been primarily doing for as long as I could remember: reeling and reacting.

the miracle

Anyone with an eating disorder occasionally doubts his or her own sanity. If you're bulimic, you literally can't stop thinking about food, and you don't care if your stomach is stretching. There's an uncontrollable force inside you demanding that you eat. And the doctors had never told me that it wasn't my fault. Instead, they gave me diets to stick to and told me about the great rewards of self-control. So when I started reading about nutrients proven to normalize cravings and blood sugar, I began to question some of my own harsh self-judgments. After a little more than a week on these supplements, my cravings and even the sedative effect and mood problems that followed my binges began to diminish.

There was also another unexpected benefit to my new regimens: my skin was changing. Since high school, I'd depended on hydrocortisone ointment for my flaking red chin and eyelids and "extra, extra dry" skin creams for my painfully parched legs and torso. I thought my skin problems were the hand I'd been dealt for the long haul. But one day as I reached for my lotion, I realized my skin wasn't screaming. There was no itch. And I hadn't had a rash since about a month after I started my liver regimen, which included essential fatty acid supplements. It was a miracle. My belief in natural substances was galvanized.

Experiencing such incredible physical improvement with so little work seemed like I was getting away with something. Applying the new things I learned wasn't work. I never felt guilty, inadequate, or resentful like I had when forcing myself to stick to "good" behavior in the past. The more I learned, the more I felt like I was indulging in secret decadent beauty splurges only I understood. My positive actions based on this powerful new knowledge began to overshadow my negative self-doubt. I felt stirrings of self-respect as I began to build myself up from nothing, one informed choice at a time.

As the weeks went by, I added more supplements to improve my metabolism and mood, and they made a difference. When I should have gained weight, it stayed the same, and when it should have stayed the same, I lost weight. For the first time since I moved to New York, I felt that I would soon overcome my disease. But as the weeks went by, I still continued to binge, though less frequently and usually with less consequence. The fake, packaged, hydrogenated food and diet soda were replaced with mounds of whole-grain breads, nut butters, and real (non-hydrogenated) desserts. I was still beating myself up but with boxing gloves on. My ever-accumulating knowledge about food and health left me no more room to rationalize. I knew exactly what I was doing to myself, but I just could not stop. I began to resign myself to my disease—until that night when I wrote that final desperate journal entry and gave up my when-I-get-thin dreams for good and pledged to love my body and myself, even if I failed.

the transformation

Without exercising or changing my diet, I started to lose weight. I can't tell you how many pounds I lost each week since I never looked at a scale, but the loss was steady. The change was even more evident to my colleagues in the fashion world and to my own family.

"How are you doing this?" everyone asked, "It must take discipline and willpower." It was almost impossible to explain that I wasn't following any rules and that I was eating what I wanted. I was no longer compelled to eat when I wasn't hungry, and if I was busy, I could even forget to eat, which *never* could have happened before. At the same time, I was truly tasting and enjoying food more than I ever had before.

A slow and sustained weight loss continued for the next three years. My body stopped shrinking at a size 6—down from my former size 18. I had no idea where I was going or what I could look or feel like. Still focused on my health, looking beautiful was the last thing on my mind.

I never considered myself to be particularly gullible, but it hit me at one point during that shrinking phase that most of the choices I'd been making all my life—which I'd assumed were the *only* choices—had been defined, if not dictated, by the food and beauty industries. I started paying attention to information I had ignored before, such as overseas studies and clusters of small independent studies, simply because they weren't reported on the five o'clock news. I was deeply humbled by how truthful this information felt and how its value continued to manifest itself in my own body. I couldn't understand why virtually all of what I'd been reading had been passed over in TV health segments and government-funded research. (This was the early 1990s, mind you.) I wanted to know why information with the potential to help so many people was not being talked about. Why did I have to go through what I did, risk my health, waste my disposable income, and forfeit my quality of life if there existed proven therapies or therapies with potential rewards that could at least be tried without risk of serious side effects?

the truth

As I read explanation after explanation, fact after fact, and law after law, consensus among doctors—even traditionally trained Ivy League doctors who were beginning to combine the best of conventional and natural healing in their own practices—was clear: the natural, therapeutic substances that had been at the foundation of my healing and transformation may work, but they don't fit into the healthcare industry in a profitable (patentable) way and are therefore either ignored or subjected to biased scrutiny.

I was stunned to realize that there must be countless therapeutic substances no one was hearing about but also irreversibly intrigued and more hopeful for the future—at least my own future—than ever before. In fact, somehow understanding why some of the best information would never be thrust in front of me on billboards or in my favorite magazines made all of my new discoveries that much more valuable to me.

I started to view everything differently. Television ads. Billboards. Government guidelines. It was as if a filter that had been deadening my senses—and sensibilities—for most of my life was being removed layer by layer. The more I learned about how foods, cosmetics, and drugs were made, tested, and regulated, the more I wanted to go out on the street with a megaphone, post notices, and shake people.

I stopped following diet and beauty trends and began to make informed choices based solely on the proven benefit, potency, and purity of my products and regimens. My purchases were no longer dictated by ads and social approval but rather by my *body's* approval. I became keenly aware of the difference between expensive, high-end packaging and the actual quality of a product. I was no longer sold on products that merely *contained* good ingredients but came to seek products that were also free of known irritants. And that was the difference between my own criterion and that of everyone else I knew at that time. Soon I was buying the highest-quality cosmetics and enjoying results I knew even the "privileged" were not aware of.

new priorities

I soon found myself spending more money on whole foods, supplements, and non-irritating beauty products than on manicures and shoes. And if I temporarily reverted to my old habits because access to my new preferences was limited (like when I visited my hometown), then the old cravings and physical agitations returned, reminding me why I'd switched to a purer path.

By age twenty-six, my beauty began to unfold and I glimpsed nature's intention in the mirror for the first time. At thirty, I looked younger than I had when I was twenty. I saw a different person altogether. One day when

I washed off my elaborate makeup job I suddenly realized that I had an innate beauty that shouldn't be covered up. I soon realized that I had the potential to be one of those women who could get away with wearing little or no makeup. I was stunned. My joy in being a woman began to emerge for the first time.

As for all those models who once seemed like a different species, today I understand who the alien really was. For twelve years *I* had been an alien to nature's intention for me. When I began writing this book, it was more than nine years since the final breakthrough that changed the physical and emotional course of my life. I haven't weighed myself in over ten years, but I'm still the same size 6. I don't really work out at a gym, but I do like to move and I do things I had never dreamed I would do, like ski and rollerblade. I dart up the stairs effortlessly now because my body feels good and my cells are happy and well cared for. I don't deny myself any particular food—except fake foods, which no longer hold any appeal for me. I haven't heard the word "should" in my head regarding food since that night it all finally clicked. Amazingly, what I desire seems to have become one and the same with what makes me feel and look good. It's like "beauty nirvana."

you don't need a crisis to be transformed

What I have come to realize is that how I once treated myself was not just a result of my eating disorder; it was also a result of our culture and the images and advertising ceaselessly thrust in front of me. For so many years I was in a holding pattern, and each time I started over, I dragged along the same stubborn mind-sets about how to live and how to achieve my body and beauty goals while lacking the same crucial information. These deeply ingrained beliefs muffled my instincts, my sensibilities, and my own criteria for what I put on and in my body. It took a crisis to challenge the myths and my unhealthy views to enable me to move in a new direction.

As I look around me today, I see a potential in most people that they may not yet dare imagine for themselves. And I know it is within their reach. When you start where I did, the effects of the "makeup-less makeover" are particularly dramatic. But by sharing what I learned the hard way, I hope to empower you to avoid the crisis and wasted years on futile, misguided attempts to look and feel better. If someone had shared with me what I will share with you in this book, I might have lived my teens in my teens rather than in my twenties and thirties!

Chapter 2

the PROCESS OF SHEDDING

People ask me: What did you do differently the day you started losing weight? But I had begun no diet, no fitness plan, no deprivation, and no drugs. I wasn't transformed by losing weight, and amazingly, I didn't lose weight by setting out to become thin. I had no beauty or weight goals or plans when the pounds started coming off. In fact, my transformation didn't start or end with weight loss. My real beauty story started when I let go of all my beauty goals. My real process of "shedding" was about shedding the stubborn mind-sets, my relationship with food, and the burdens that had denatured my life and kept my beauty from emerging.

The truth is that beauty and comfort in our own skin and bodies is a *natural, effortless state* that is too often thrown off-balance by modern assaults, conveniences, and toxins to which our bodies are unable to adapt.

sometimes it's what you *don't* do that makes you beautiful

Beauty is not about buying, applying, and doing all the "right" things. It is what remains in all of us once we lift away the burdens and stop the self-sabotage that prevents it from thriving. I used to spend hours in front of the mirror without taking in the true state of my beauty. For all those years, it had been obscured, not only by layers of makeup, wardrobe "noise," and products but also by a lifetime of built-up, compensatory, and distractive measures and layers of false beliefs I'd adopted on how to achieve my physical goals. As I shed these mind-sets and self-sabotaging practices one by one, I was able to re-attune to my own true essence, and I could hear the long-muffled messages from my body that had been there all along.

Before we begin to cultivate our true radiance, we must first recover and reconnect with it by lifting away the barriers that stand in its way. If you've gotten yourself caught up in a merry-go-round of problem-causing self-care strategies, you can't keep accumulating products and practices and expect to be transformed. You must first recognize the assaults and then stop them, reverse them, and recover from them in order to reclaim your true potential and take off in a new direction.

This most critical step toward vitality, which I call "shedding," is a cyclical journey of undoing, uncovering, and unveiling. In the following chapters, I'll take you through a process of shedding the self-limiting mind-sets, toxins, and misguided beauty and lifestyle rituals you may have accumulated over the years. Each assault you shed is beauty in the bank, and each pro-beauty lifestyle upgrade will yield generous immediate and long-term dividends.

Because the solutions in the chapters ahead have far more appeal and power to reward and uplift you than the second-rate substitutions or unappealing choices you may have tried to adopt in the past, you shouldn't think of these exciting new choices as substitutions at all. Think of them as upgrades. Upgrading your regimens is both joyful and self-motivating.

the process of shedding brings deeper issues to the surface

As more and more layers of outer sensory irritation, distraction, and blinders are stripped away, deeper chemical and emotional issues that have been thriving on and driving their most stubborn habits and vices may begin to emerge at the surface with new transparency. By continuing the process of shedding, you can literally starve these emotional and chemical roots of the unhealthy acts and substances that keep them alive, and loosen their grip. Shedding is the best way to break free of the downward cycle of self-sabotage.

As each cycle of upgrades and recovery leads to the next, you'll rise far above that old merry-go-round in an upward spiral toward a thriving state that glows of nature's intention.

each cycle of shedding is greater than the sum of its parts

Each area of your life affects the others. As you apply the principles of shedding to one area, you'll find it is only a matter of time before it migrates to others. As your knowledge, self-respect, and ability to think independently increase, your outer beauty practices will simplify. Some will be shed entirely.

The spiritual rewards of shedding are as profound and exciting as the physical ones. Giving up the numbing false comforts of conventional beauty routines and embracing powerful new choices that resonate with your long-neglected, better instincts not only restores your well-being but also your soul. With each cycle of beauty recovery, you'll feel a new burden lift away, and you will soon come to realize just how weighed-down and denatured the old you had become.

From this foundation you will be fully primed to reap the maximum rewards of feeding, cultivating, and rebuilding your beauty in a whole new way with the most amazing substances and strategies.

there's beauty in the truth: shed the mind-sets that keep you stuck

The process of shedding starts inside our heads. By simply reading the previous pages, your process has already begun. But it's easy to underestimate the invisible barriers that can paralyze our progress or blind our sensibilities to real solutions, even when we think our minds are open. None of us likes to believe it, but much of how we treat ourselves and what we have become has been determined by our acceptance of the information, images, and choices we are bombarded with every day. Until we see them through new eyes, we will continue to be misled. By looking at some of the myths that keep us in a holding pattern, I hope to light a clearer path as I guide you up the spiral. Let me start with a few of the most pervasive myths.

> *MYTH: **Beauty requires willpower and self-discipline.***
>
> *TRUTH: **Willpower and self-discipline are dead-end roads.***

Willpower and self-discipline require us to disconnect from ourselves and treat ourselves impersonally and unnaturally. They are damage-control measures that stand in for real solutions to unexplored issues. They can be applied to any kind of regimen with the same disconnecting result. From the way you approach a zit—search and destroy!—to the way you approach your weight issue, the drill sergeant's attitude is the kind we often commit to at the dermatologist's office or on New Year's Day. Willpower can even be applied with disastrous results, as demonstrated by the will to skip meals and destroy your own metabolism in the process. While exciting in its extremity and even effective at first, it almost certainly leads to disappointment and compounded problems. The greatest risk in the outside-in, bulldozer, show-your-body-who's boss approach—which I also call the "do-something" impulse—is that it lures and distracts us with short-sighted rewards as it keeps us from identifying the real problems and solutions, which should never require us to drive or deprive ourselves.

Quitting cold turkey, adding more reps, eating rice cakes, or exfoliating our poor skin 24/7 are often the damage control measures we must depend on until we resolve the real emotional, chemical, and logistical issues that feed our problems. Strict regimens and inflexible tactics will never make us beautiful in the long run, and they are dangerous substitutes for authentic needs. They may take pounds off or temporarily smooth our complexion, but they will leave us off-kilter and unhealthy and distract us from other lingering issues that need attention.

Here's the good news: It is entirely possible to reap unprecedented rewards *without* frustration and setbacks. I don't believe in deprivation or drills. I've learned that what's good for you can be pleasurable, powerful, and transforming. All you need are better *tools* so you can make more inspired and effective choices.

don't force your beauty—support it

The process of shedding is a gentle, kind one. It is never forced, and it compels itself with joyful, harmonious momentum at each stage. After leaving behind the old harsh approaches, you'll all but forget the discomforts and confusion you left behind—that is, until you try living like you used to for a day. You won't believe what you've been putting yourself through! We are far too harsh with ourselves. We hire face-sanders and commando fitness trainers; we exercise epic willpower to skip meals; we fight to show our hair, our sweat glands, and any other natural part of us who's boss, while underestimating our body's own healing and regulating mechanisms and ignoring our own emotional issues and body chemistry. On top of all that we pass ceaseless judgment on our reflections in the mirror.

As you embark on the journey ahead, allow yourself to forget every preconceived notion you've ever had about being beautiful, staying healthy, or getting fit. Suspend judgment and open yourself to a world of new possibilities.

Here are a few of the more controversial ideas you will become familiar with as you continue:

- Forcing yourself to exercise when you really hate it may only be a crutch you must rely on until you face the real issues that weigh you down. By correcting your mood, food, and hormonal issues, you'll find your body will *want* to move.
- Harsh skin regimens won't give you the most beautiful skin in the long run. To regain your most glowing skin, you must help it recover its own pro-beauty and anti-aging functions.
- Fighting or denying your sweet tooth is no longer necessary for a beautiful body. Handling your cravings with the new sweet alternatives that don't assault your body will allow you to feel satisfied, get healthier, and change your shape at the same time.
- You needn't beat yourself up because quitting a bad habit cold turkey didn't stick. Attacking your vice, which is merely a symptom, won't help. Starving it of its chemical, ideological, and logistical support system through shedding is the road map to real and permanent freedom.

The painless way is often the healthiest and smartest way. Real solutions rarely require anything more than the transformational tools I will share with you in the next chapter and then help you apply in the chapters that follow.

It sounds almost too good to be true, but the best solutions cause no setbacks, guilt trips, and new problems that require high-tech maintenance. They won't make you feel guilty, inadequate, or resentful like the other ways of "being good." These techniques—which you'll find are so easy that they feel like cheating—are actually a part of the most natural, healthy, and intuitive approach there is. Best of all, a successful inside-out approach will make the rest of you more beautiful, too.

> **MYTH: *Beauty is a frivolous pursuit.***
>
> **TRUTH: *Beauty reflects your quality of life.***
>
> Some of us may be genetically predisposed to hearty physical and even mental constitutions, but none of us are invulnerable to the ravages of time, or worse, the toxic hazards on planet Earth. Even lucky folks need to deftly navigate today's harsh new landscape if lifelong radiance is the goal. Such a goal is neither shallow nor trivial since beauty and vitality are inextricably connected to health and quality of life. To achieve them requires awareness and a strong connection with one's inner voice and purpose.
>
> Beauty is not a frivolous issue, nor is it a vanity issue. It is a quality-of-life issue and a birthright we tend to forfeit far too easily by turning opportunities to *create* ourselves into mundane regimens by which we merely maintain ourselves—or worse yet, let others maintain us.
>
> We attempt to fix or improve ourselves by becoming customers of industry-prompted regimens that cause new problems. We've lapsed in our discernment of the raw materials we use to care for ourselves. With

all of our comforts and gadgetry, too many of us are deprived of the joys in the simpler things: the joy in body and spirit that can make living of modest means more rewarding than living with every material advantage money can buy; the joy of connection with our own glowing essence; the joy of priceless vitality. Vitality *is* the universal beauty aesthetic.

you've created what you are today; only you can create what you become tomorrow

As much as I was a victim of the ceaseless suggestions that perpetuated my self-sabotage, only *I* was ultimately responsible for it, and nothing or no one could have made me change until I took charge of healing myself.

Though I regularly refer to the dubious information and negative messages that we are all bombarded with, make no mistake: You have created what you are today, with varying degrees of help from countless influences. Today you will create what you will be tomorrow. There's no point in blaming irresponsible companies, unresponsive politicians, or the "system" for the problems of the world around us that have invaded our lives and our beauty. Relying on social, cultural, or commercial cues for our choices is what causes us to stray from our better instincts in the first place. If you start sentences with "My doctor has me taking this" or "My trainer has me doing that," stop yourself. Only *you* have *yourself* doing whatever it is you choose to do. Stop following and start setting your own course.

What I never learned in beauty school or with any doctor, weight-loss counselor, or nutritionist was the importance of masterminding my own transformation by getting informed and rejecting self-defeating motivations to win the battles of chemistry, culture, and convenience. Only we can transform ourselves, and we must identify and cultivate our assets and discern our raw materials with the passion of an artist.

the REAL TOOLS FOR TRANSFORMATION

The real tools for transformation transcend trends and technology to help us achieve the vitality that the most sophisticated hair and makeup techniques can only mimic. These tools—which took me more than a decade to stumble on—will save you the needless struggle and the dangers of hitting bottom, so you can begin your own *real* transformation today. They can free you from the assault–recovery merry-go-round and break through all your beauty glass ceilings. If any of the following tools are missing from any beauty, body, or self-help approach, success will eventually crumble.

By applying these tools throughout the journey ahead, you'll have unprecedented inspiration and support for what might otherwise require a blind leap of faith—which is exactly what I want to discourage—and needless inconvenience.

tool #1: the magic motivation

Think Health and Beauty Will Follow

I learned the hard way that profound transformation doesn't happen unless the right motivation is in place. Vanity-based pursuits can be effective distractions from the real issues that keep us stuck. To be sexually appealing, look good for the lingerie shoot, win the role, and be lean and mean for the corporate machine are all motivations that keep us at war with ourselves, no matter how "successfully" we change our exterior because they do not address our essential needs. Superficial goals lead to superficial measures and to superficial results that must be maintained through ongoing struggles with willpower and self-discipline. Motivations of self-love and health, on the other hand, work with and never undermine our sense of self-worth, and they engage our self-preservation instinct whereas other motivations trample it.

The most profound journey to radiance begins when we give up beauty goals and focus instead on health. The vanity motive dies hard, but what dies with it are the self-destructive, drastic measures we had mistakenly thought would bring us the greatest and quickest rewards.

Beauty and Self-Preservation

The survival instinct is a primitive instinct we can sometimes allow to atrophy in our cushy, civilized world. My self-preservation instinct was the final motivator within me as I reached my health crisis, and once it kicked in, its power took me by surprise. The self-preservation instinct fully engages both instinct and intellect. It inspires a material vigilance that can guide countless superior choices and bear untold fruit if we let it lead the way, even if we haven't reached a crisis. Survival is as much an issue today as it was in the time when we faced sabre-toothed tigers, only the threats today are far less obvious.

Acting on aesthetic or external physical goals with a primary focus on impressing or being accepted by others will leave holes and leaks in both our souls and our commitments to ourselves. This is why it is incredibly hazardous to enter into any field or social sphere in which success is contingent on looks. If achieving the physical standard is anything but courtesy of incredible genes or very high self-esteem, then we've got a recipe for emotional and physical problems if we set out to get there by someone else's terms, time frames, or standards, which we often quickly adopt.

I've seen both the frustration and the danger that models go through when they don't even have the luxury of putting their own health before the constant pressure to be the size that is printed on their promo cards. Many women, particularly young women, feel almost the same degree of pressure. In the name of beauty, they purge, starve themselves, smoke, and undergo liposuction. Many do damage control by consuming empty foods that throw their body's chemistry further off-balance, which leads to more bingeing.

In my work, I have observed that the plus-size model who takes care of herself has the healthiest self-image. But women who are large because they're abusing themselves rarely feel good about themselves, no matter how many well-meaning organizations tell them that being large is OK. Yes, we must love ourselves, no matter how we look, and maybe that's a reason to listen to what our looks tell us. Beyond our weight or size or how good our makeup, hair, and wardrobe looks, we can learn so much from the mirror and by listening to our bodies.

Your Health Is the Most Rational Passion There Is

Our society accepts sports and car fanatics. We prize the successful pursuit of the perfect bikini wax. But those who carefully evaluate what they put on and in their bodies are often met with attitude or harassment in some circles. Caring about our health doesn't make us fanatics. It makes us rational and conscious. To be passive about health is to be lacking in self-respect and taking for granted our own capacity for beauty and happiness.

Just as our spirit affects our beauty, our health affects both spirit and beauty directly. An alarming number of people in developed countries increasingly develop obesity problems, diabetes, heart disease, high blood pressure, and various cancers—most of which have been shown to be largely preventable with healthy habits. Even genetic predispositions are not necessarily the final word since science has discovered that the expression of certain genes can sometimes be overridden or delayed by lifestyle factors. With this knowledge, it is irrational not to take advantage of this information and take painless steps to ensure your most precious vitality.

Aim Higher than the Mirror or the Scale

Most people see a nutritionist, trainer, or doctor for matters of appearance or relief of a symptom. But suppose you went to these specialists to improve your health. For example, you might really throw off your dermatologist if you use him as part of your plan to get or stay healthy. Imagine going in only for a comprehensive diagnosis to get to the cause. Imagine making your doctor aware of your other symptoms and your history, asking him to consider the possible side effects your habits or prescription drugs may be causing, and swatting his hands each time he reached for the prescription pad or a free sample of steroid cream.

Sometimes even your doctor isn't operating on the best information or motivations. For example, it's one thing to diet down or take a potentially dangerous drug to achieve a healthy weight; it's quite another to focus on getting healthy and drop the excess weight in the process. I have never heard of this approach being advocated by a conventional doctor, but it's the healthiest, most successful, and most painless approach of all.

Similarly, the most effective motivations to exercise go beyond weight loss. If you focus instead on its antidepressant, stress-busting, and bone-strengthening effects, then the attitude you'll adopt toward exercise is more likely to uplift you rather than make you feel self-conscious, resentful, or judgmental of yourself for falling short of your physical goals. There's nothing negative about a 100 percent healthy motivation!

Aim higher for yourself. And make sure that the professionals who advise your choices are aiming high enough for you, too.

MYTH: *A hard body is the healthiest body.*

TRUTH: *Cellular health is what counts.*

A heavy person can be healthier and more radiant than a hard body (though the healthier you are, the harder it is to stay heavy). How healthy you are on a *cellular* level determines your vitality and how much you feel like moving. It also shows in your face, your hair texture, and your sense of well-being, not to mention your doctor's blood tests.

It is possible to be a healthy weight and be far less healthy than someone whose weight is considered too high. A mother may keep more weight off in the long run with less struggle and healthier results by chasing her two-year-old around than by joining an aerobics class. But being guilted into thinking she should add a workout to her already physically demanding day keeps her from facing the emotional, chemical, and hormonal issues that affect her weight. Give up the mind-set that a beautiful shape is about sweat or that a cut body is always the healthiest body. While regular activity is important and can help make you beautiful, your shape and even your desire to move is largely affected by your nutrient and hormone balance and the vitality of your cells. The beauty you exude glows from your cells, not from your muscles.

In the name of beauty, focus on your health. Change your New Year's resolutions from weight to targeted health goals, like "stabilize my blood sugar," "get my metabolism back," "balance my moods and cravings," "close my nutrition deficits," or "clear up my digestive problems." Beauty payoffs will follow once these health goals are set.

Summary
- Think *health* and beauty will follow.
- Superficial goals lead to superficial means and superficial results.
- Trade in the thin and sexy goals. The vanity motive isn't the place to start. You need the power of the magic motive: health.
- Celebrate your beauty as it emerges but be motivated by health.

tool #2: complete information

The More You Know, the Better You Live and Look

As powerful as it is, the health motive can only take you so far if you are limited by incomplete information. If you rely on TV health reports and other sources currently sponsored by food, body-care, and drug companies, you're not getting the whole story. And believe me, we all need the unsponsored information we haven't been getting.

Even if we apply our best instincts to our choices, there's a need for a heightened awareness in today's world. Unnatural circumstances require a measure of vigilance that goes beyond the intuitive. Only we can protect ourselves from the beauty wildcards—environmental toxins, agricultural experiments, untested chemical combinations, and hormone impostors our bodies have never had to deal with in the past. We can take steps to minimize the impact of these wildcards only if we are aware of them.

New World, New Tools: Why Instinct Is Not Enough Today

A hundred years ago, when unprocessed foods, clean water, and truly fresh air were commonplace, becoming informed might have been more of a luxury than a necessity. You could pretty much learn what was good for you by listening to your grandma. But our mothers' generation may have been the last for which basic beauty advice could suffice. "Eat right, drink enough water, exercise, get your beauty sleep, and get plenty of sunshine" may have been enough back then, but life has become more dangerous in ways that aren't always obvious. Conventional beauty wisdom is no match for our modern beauty challenges. Even our instincts fail to detect the new risks. In order to thrive—not merely survive—in today's world, we've got to re-hone and re-inform our beauty instincts to navigate the changing landscape.

In this increasingly toxic age, the products—and particularly the remedies we use—merit greater skepticism than many of us are willing to give. It has also become increasingly clear that we cannot count on government regulation and guidelines to protect our best interests. It is more important than ever to expand our information horizons and approach our beauty with greater care. And though unglamorous truths can be disturbing at first, acting on them can knock down the biggest barriers that keep us from our true, vital potential.

Good Information Replaces Hard Work

It doesn't take hard work or deprivation to end dry skin or cravings; it just takes information. For example, it isn't painful to install a water filter in your shower that will spare your skin—and the rest of your body—premature aging while making your hair silkier. It's not work to take a supplement that reduces varicose veins or to upgrade a harmful product to a proven alternative. Complete information can lay to rest the myths and rationalizations that have kept you from thriving. It spares you all kinds of "rides" and puts you on a different playing field that transcends privilege and social standing. Favoring beauty-sparing, nontoxic approaches to health and beauty are the result of getting informed.

Becoming Your Own Best Expert Is Easier than You Think

Most people put off getting informed, and I can't blame them. Unless you have easy access to sources of complete, unfiltered information, it can be a chore to dig it up. My goal is to spare you the searching and give you a healthy infusion of the facts, strategies, and resources you haven't been getting so you can become an expert in what's best for you in a very short time.

For example, after familiarizing yourself with the proven nutritional options for improving your specific skin condition, you may, after one sitting, know more about cultivating good skin than you'll ever learn from a dermatologist. Western medicine has traditionally positioned itself as the all-knowing source of health information, but it is still almost exclusively about curing symptoms, not about health-supporting solutions or achieving vitality. However, if you make the decision to learn for yourself what is best for you, the result will not only be liberating clarity and utter simplicity but also a far more beautiful future. It is within all of us to become our own best expert and advocate. If we don't, no one else will.

Get the Straight Science: Beauty Shouldn't Require Blind Faith

Most people would like to *think* they could get beautiful without harsh skin regimens, drugs, or epic willpower, but they don't believe it. I know what it means to be resistant and skeptical. Despite my belief in the solutions I've uncovered, I don't automatically believe that what works for one person will work for another. As an informed layman, I advocate skepticism and discourage blind faith. I also believe it is important to point out that science is there for the people, but it is not always reported. Science shouldn't be left to industry interpretation or "professional use only." In the years since I first started investigating the importance of alternative beauty and health strategies and nontoxic products, the body of scientific evidence that validates them has been growing by leaps and bounds. As our unnatural world and products cause the average person—which no longer includes you, since you are reading this book!—to develop more unnatural health and beauty syndromes that traditional medicine cannot solve, society's interest in natural solutions will continue to grow. The key is to get hooked up to the stream of unfiltered information that can complete the whole—not just the familiar—picture of your options right now as the science—and even the anecdotal evidence that generally precedes it—unfolds.

Are You an Obedient Consumer?

Whether we think we are gullible or not, as naturally trusting beings, marketing deceptions have had an impact on our lives. By accepting as truth what we hear most often, what comes in the most appealing package, or what is endorsed by most medical spokespeople, we too often reward the companies that spend their millions on everything but the actual product. Appealing poetry, packaging, and virtual smells and tastes distract us from the actual substances we're being sold. And to keep us off the trail to any truths we're not meant to discover, every effort is made to keep consumers from demanding the details: "Trust us. We're the professionals." "You don't understand the science." "It's more complicated than that." "You don't have the facts." "It's best to go ahead with the conventional approach." "Take control and take this..." "It's the number-one recommended choice." Don't let anyone shame or distract you from demanding details, reading the small print, and becoming the only expert you need to trust. Remember: Science is there for everyone. Don't be a "good" customer; be a discerning connoisseur.

Patents Equal Profits: The Catch-22 That's Been Keeping You in the Dark

Unadulterated forms of natural substances cannot be patented, and therefore they don't make companies the kind of profits patented drugs and beauty products can. Many supplements and herbal remedies have been shown to have healing or protective effects at much lower costs and with

MYTH: **The media will keep me informed.**

TRUTH: **The media is not a source of balanced information.**

The published science that verifies natural approaches is often overlooked by the media due to the industry support that patented, money-making drugs get but natural alternatives don't. Loosening of media regulation in the 1990s led to the rapid consolidation of media control into the hands of the mighty few corporations who now handle the nation's entire broadcast media industry. Talk-show health segments are often sponsored by pharmaceutical companies. These inherent conflicts of interest mean that most people's primary sources of information have lost their basic pillars of objectivity. We are living in a new era of industry-owned information flow and even industry-owned and -influenced science.

We can no longer become informed by the average news report or magazine story. Even though many important stories regarding your health and beauty do make it to prime time, they are often understated or quickly upstaged if the money-making potential is not there. Stories like those on the benefits of supplements or the dangers of antibacterial soaps get lost due to lack of industry sponsorship. Consequently, not only do we not hear about lots of products that work, but perhaps of even more concern, we also don't always hear about some of the dangers of what we currently eat, take, and apply.

For the same reason, research discrediting nondrug treatments often garners wide attention, even when it might only be one negative—and perhaps poorly designed—study out of dozens of underreported positive ones. Though not a beauty product, one clear example of this skewed media coverage is the attack leveled at the herb St. John's wort, a natural (read: unpatentable) substance shown in at least twenty-five double-blind clinical studies to effectively treat mild to moderate depression. But what most of the public heard about was one study that found it failed to alleviate *severe* depression, a condition for which it has never been historically used or intended. This study was funded by Pfizer, a pharmaceutical company whose own drugs are not considered effective against severe depression when used alone, according to the Merck Manual guidelines and the Herb Research Foundation. Whether natural substances or pharmaceutical drugs are the best treatment for a given condition is something only a patient and a doctor can decide together, but the point is that with the current media mechanics, the American public is far more likely to hear about the news that benefits the industries that contribute funds for air time.

fewer side effects than the corresponding drugs. Yet without the quantifiable financial payoff that patent protection affords—which pays for the glamorous ad campaigns, the TV health segments, and even some of the celebrities who mention drug treatments on the air during casual interviews—there is little corporate interest in funding natural substances for the expensive clinical trials required for Food and Drug Administration (FDA) approval. Furthermore, the $500,000-plus price tag of FDA approval is far out of the range of most sellers of natural substances, which, because their product can't be patented, can therefore never recoup such an investment. Keep this in mind as you view billboards, advertisements, and TV health segments and as you peruse the decidedly un-slick aisles of a natural products store.

It is also important to know that pharmaceutical and chemical industries are in the habit of developing synthetic—and therefore patentable—versions of effective natural substances and then marketing them to the public as the best or only existing treatment or solution. For example, scientists are now working to create an anti-breast-cancer drug they have synthesized from the natural substance sulforaphane, a component of broccoli. The patented version, called oxomate, may be available in several years, but sulforaphane has been available as a supplement for years. A related substance from broccoli called I3C—also currently available as a supplement—has been shown to inhibit the growth of certain human breast-cancer cells better than the drug tamoxifen under laboratory conditions without the side effects that have made tamoxifen so controversial. While you probably haven't heard about I3C, much pharmaceutical-grade advertisement, media fanfare, and inflated costs will likely come with the announcement of oxomate.

Similarly, the manufacture of progestin was the product of the goal to synthesize a patentable (profitable) form of progesterone from foods like wild yam and soy, which have often been publicly ridiculed and dismissed by the very industry that scrambled to synthesize them. Incidentally, the synthetic hormone showed immediate evidence of possible serious side effects, while the natural, bio-identical hormone produced none.

MYTH: *My doctor will keep me informed.*

TRUTH: *Your doctor may not know about or consider natural treatment options.*

Many doctors are too busy and—believe it—not *required* to look at independent research in medical journals for new treatment options. Some doctors depend entirely on pharmaceutical sales reps for ongoing treatment information. Pharmaceutical companies have historically spent upwards of $13,000 per doctor per year to court physicians with ceaseless perks and incentives, like frequent flyer miles, Broadway shows, exotic trips, and free gas fill-ups, to sell drugs. They have also sent rebates to pharmacists and insurance-claims representatives as encouragement to favor their drugs. Courting your doctor and the media is expensive business, and unpatentable natural product manu-facturers could not begin to compete, even if the establishment were in their favor.

Even *science* is no longer sacred. Scientists are currently allowed to accept money or stock from a company while conducting research on its products. When the government attempted to impose restrictions on these conflicts of interest, industry lobby prevailed. According to several articles in the *New York Times*, scientific misconduct is a result of these conflicts. One FDA official was quoted as saying that it has got-ten "completely out of control."

A review of literature and interviews conducted by Dr. Thomas S. Bodenheimer of the University of California, San Francisco, concluded that when drug companies paid for a trial of a new drug, "biases can be, and have been, intentionally introduced that favor the company funding the study."

Kind of a brain twister, isn't it? Isn't unbiased study the very foun-dation of science? Are we to put scientists, doctors, or any other pro-fessionals or politicians in a category of honesty or invulnerability to corruption over anyone else? If not, then why are these conflicts allowed? Don't expect an answer anytime soon. In the meantime, the informed choices you make will send a powerful message to the indus-tries that have come to exploit such conflicts.

DID YOU BUY THESE EXPERIMENTS?

These controversial diet and personal-care products have been hotly debated because of their possible negative effects on the body. If you bought these products, it's probably because you were told they were safe. But did you get to hear both sides of the debate? Here are some widespread medical views that were mostly lost in the media due to lack of corporate sponsorship.

- **Wow potato chips and other Olestra-containing products:** Several countries, including Canada, denied approval of Olestra as a food ingredient because it blocks the absorption of crucial fat-soluble vitamins.

- **Antibacterial soaps:** Like antibiotics, these soaps destroy both good and bad bacteria and could give rise to microbes that are resistant to such products.

- **Nutrasweet/aspartame:** Routine consumption of aspartame-containing products may create a build-up of methanol in the body, leading to neurological and other problems.

- **Fat-free foods:** The well-known consequence of high-glycemic foods—as fat-free foods tend to be—is that they raise triglycerides and can lead to insulin problems, unhealthy blood-sugar metabolism, weight gain, and even diabetes.

GOVERNMENT GUIDELINES AND REGULATIONS: TOO LITTLE TOO LATE

- For years fat-free recommendations from government scientists were based largely on speculation and conflicted with common medical knowledge about the actions of insulin.

- As early as 1979 reports indicated the dangers of phenylpropanolamine, an ingredient in diet pills and cold remedies. But it wasn't pulled from the shelves until 2000, and not before it caused needless strokes in hundreds of healthy people.

- Fenfluramine-phentermine (Fen-Phen) was formerly an ingredient of anti-obesity drugs, such as Redux and Pondimin. Many doctors prescribed these drugs without fully disclosing the risk of heart and lung problems. According to FDA statements as well as a Mayo Clinic study published in the August 28, 1997, *New England Journal of Medicine*, as many as one-third of users studied showed heart abnormalities by the time the drug was recalled in 1997.

- Putting a cosmetic on the market does not require safety data on ingredients or any pre-market review, and manufacturers do not have to report consumer complaints from their cosmetics. Currently, cosmetics can only be regulated once they appear in the marketplace. Of all cosmetic chemicals used, nearly nine hundred are toxic, according to the National Institute of Occupational Safety and Health.

- The Environmental Protection Agency (EPA) has found traces of shampoos, antibiotics, hormones, and chemicals from drug and personal-care products in rivers and waterways all over the United States, and yet it has made no long-term plans for cleanup or restrictions as other countries have begun to do.

- According to documents examined by two researchers at the University of California, San Francisco, in the 1980s and early 1990s, tobacco companies successfully exerted pressure on pharmaceutical companies to tone down ad campaigns for products aimed to help people kick their smoking habits.
- American studies that showed cholesterol-raising effects from tropical palm-kernel oil, which have influenced our fat choices for decades, may have been done using common oxidized, refined, or otherwise adulterated oil (the nature of the oils was not revealed in the American studies); however, studies done in Malaysia, the native source of raw, fresh palm-kernel oil, showed palm-kernel oil to actually lower cholesterol levels.

The Ultimate Beauty Secret: A Healthy Dose of Disenchantment

Unfortunately, the search for complete information inevitably leads to the shocking revelation that some companies we all grew up trusting are, in fact, led by quite a different set of motives. I encourage you to think critically and never assume that a treatment, product, or food is safe or good for you just because your grandmother did.

Corporations that damage the environment and harm us can still run the most heartwarming ads and employ good, upstanding—though perhaps misled—people. Good doctors, scientists, and farmers of conscience can still serve as unwitting pawns to industries. When the hands-on people—from repairmen to doctors—we're taught to trust aren't held accountable—or even fully informed about—their own products or services, it's easier for disconnected decision makers to do what would ordinarily seem unconscionable: put profits over people and the planet.

Fortunately, profits depend on consumers. So as a consumer, you always have the ultimate power to ask questions, demand full disclosure, or spend your dollars elsewhere. The more you know, the less you have to take anyone's word for it.

Do your body and your beauty a serious favor: Don't put your unquestioning trust in professions and industries, brand names, number-one recommended products or treatments, industry stamps of approval, or guidelines, no matter how respectable they seem. The only people you ever needed to trust entirely were your parents, and just as every parent has very human weaknesses and personal agendas, so does every regulatory agency and authority figure that influences your living choices. The sooner you let go of any remaining blind faith you have in the government's ability or incentive to protect you, the sooner you can put that faith and the role of the protector where it belongs: with *you*.

Will There Always Be a Prejudice against Alternatives?

Although many Americans now use nondrug therapies and products, the bias of the medical community and various industries continues to discourage people from exploring these options more fully. Moreover, when dealing with transgressions of any kind, purveyors of alternative treatments are dealt with far more harshly than their conventional counterparts.

For example, Dr. Alan R. Gaby, the author of the *Healthnotes Newswire* report, points out that on the numerous occasions when pharmaceutical companies have been accused of misleading advertising, the result is only a cease-and-desist order but never a confiscation of goods. In a *New Times* article, Marion Moss, a former investigator with the Texas Attorney General's office, said, "During the eight years when I was an investigator ... I had numerous occasions to work with the FDA on cases involving potential health fraud. I repeatedly saw cases against large corporations go unchallenged. Instead the agency chose to pursue cases involving alternative health care providers."

Similarly when the public tries to access information to alternative treatment through their conventional health-care providers, they often meet resistance. A 1999 University of California, San Francisco, study revealed that a vast majority of breast cancer patients incorporate alternative therapies with conventional ones but don't discuss them with their doctors. Patients cited their doctors' disinterest and lack of ability to contribute useful information among the leading reasons they kept their alternative therapies to themselves.

But even the most conservative doctors can surprise us now and then by opening their minds. In a TV interview in July 2000 Dr. Bill Fair, former chairman of urology at the prestigious Memorial Sloan-Kettering Cancer Center, was asked by NBC 4's Dr. Max Gomez, "Has the conventional medical world been arrogant in its rejection of Eastern medicine?"

Fair hesitated and then replied, "Yes, I would have to say that. I would like to think that this movement back toward more primal systems was something that originated within medicine, but it hasn't. It's the patients doing the originating. They're leading it."

Informed Choices Depend On Full Disclosure

When people are well-informed, they may choose not to use a product that hasn't been proven to be satisfactory or they may demand access to one that gives better results. Big industry is therefore well motivated to suppress negative or even inconclusive research about their own products.

Some industries have been quite successful in their efforts to keep certain information from public knowledge. For example, in the United States, the majority of people eat genetically modified foods (also known as genetically modified organisms, or GMOs) without even knowing it, much less knowing what they are. GMOs are foods that have not yet been subjected to long-term studies, have proven to be inherently unpredictable, and are considered to be potentially dangerous by many prominent scientists. Though such foods are either labeled or not allowed in Europe due to public outcry and safety concerns, in the United States they are widely sold without a label. Unless a product is 100 percent organic, which means it contains no GMOs, there is no way for consumers to know what's in their foods. Industry lobbying and pressure against laws that would require labeling and allow consumers to make informed choices are great. With regard to milk, for example, efforts have even been made by the manufacturers of the genetically modified bovine growth hormone known as rBGH to prevent dairy producers who *don't* use it from stating so explicitly on their labels. Without full disclosure, the concept of choice is merely an illusion. If we reward the actions of such shrouded industry with our uninformed patronage, we give ourselves up as guinea pigs.

MYTH: *Natural therapies are unproven.*

TRUTH: *Plenty of therapies are proven, but if they aren't patentable, you may not hear about them.*

Until the late 1990s, there was little government funding—and no pharmaceutical-industry funding—for the study of unpatentable natural substances. Public demand has begun to change that. There is now a fast-growing number of peer-reviewed, published studies confirming the benefits of hundreds of natural substances that the well-informed have known about for over a decade, other cultures have known for generations, and most doctors have scoffed at until quite recently.

> **MYTH:** *If it really worked, I would have heard about it.*
>
> **TRUTH:** *Results of important research are not always revealed to the public.*
>
> Consumers forget that the government and other social machinery are always balancing the well-being of the general public with layers of political agendas. It was long suspected but finally proven in 1999 in a stunning court ruling that the FDA had unjustly censored health claims backed by good science from appearing on nutritional supplement labels, in the name of "protecting the public." The Federal Appellate Court found that claims about the important reproductive health and birth-defect-preventing benefits of folic acid had been unconstitutionally suppressed by the FDA. For years, tens of thousands of women weren't hearing about a substance that was well documented to be crucial to their health and that of their babies. This victory over FDA bias of alternative substances has set the stage for recent legislation allowing more well-researched health claims to appear on supplement and food labels.

Declare Your Independence

Back in the days when I first discovered the supplement I needed to recover from my liver disease, the term "alternative medicine" seemed legitimate and literal. But now that natural and integrative therapies have become increasingly popular, the term is becoming outmoded.

So what do we call them if not "alternatives"? How about *informed choices*? Mainstream guidelines, mass production, and standardized care have created the alarming statistics and compromise in quality of life we hear about and experience every day. But where society has headed doesn't have to be where you're headed. Don't be another beauty statistic. Learn for yourself. Think for yourself. Don't be duped into thinking of alternatives as unproven or unpatriotic. Vote with your dollars. Demand full disclosure, good manufacturing practices, purity, choice, and real sustenance. Declare your independence from standard self-care strategies and start opening your eyes to the new world of safer, science-backed, and self-affirming solutions that are easily found by the informed consumer.

Summary

- The more you know, the better you look and live.
- Incomplete information keeps us stuck. Complete information sets us free.
- Feed your self-respect with informed acts.
- Trust solid science, your instincts, and the individuals you choose— not lab coats, professions, and industries.
- Question information that has been packaged and filtered for public consumption.
- Distinguish raw science from industry interpretation and bias.
- Demand full disclosure about everything that goes in and on your body.
- Become your own best expert. It's easier than you think.

tool #3: access to the best products and resources

Convenience Makes the Difference between Intentions and Results

All the motivation and information in the world won't help you if there's no easy way to follow through. It's important to have practical, appealing solutions in order to gain the courage to leave old mind-sets and habits behind. Living well and staying beautiful doesn't have to be difficult or expensive; it doesn't require inflexible regimens or obscure products.

Each time we simply accept the choices we feel we are stuck with, we resign ourselves to a physical destiny that nature never intended for us. There is no longer any reason for this kind of compromise. With the Internet, mail order, retailers of better products, and services popping up all

SHELF LIFE VS. QUALITY OF LIFE: AN INVERSE RELATIONSHIP

Indefinite shelf life and third-party warehousing are the backbone of mainstream food and body-care manufacturing. Removal of vital oils and biologically active components from mass-marketed foods and personal-care products and substituting them with the cheapest refined oils and fillers ensures not only the longest shelf life but also the best returns on a manufacturer's investment of raw materials. By using refined and denatured raw materials that have literally had the life sucked out of them, manufacturers not only save big on the cost of materials but also can store products indefinitely, give you quantity discounts, and still rake in the kind of profits it takes to run the most popular ad campaigns. But this win-win situation for the manufacturer is a serious loss for your beauty and quality of life.

The common thread between our souls and our physical bodies is the interconnection between ourselves and nature. Our access to pure water and biologically harmonious products, live food, and quality supplements—nature in therapeutic doses—is crucial to achieving radiance in today's denatured world.

over the country, you can now access the good life wherever you are. Living a pro-beauty lifestyle is not only practical for the first time but also far more uplifting than the standard choices we've come to accept at our own expense. You need to know and to start benefiting from the fact that today you can have it all. As you lavish these newfound delights on yourself, your definition of decadence will change completely, and your quality of life will soar.

By experimenting with the new class of superior pro-beauty products and lifestyle options presented throughout this book and in the Resources at the end, you can reset your own informed criteria for what goes on and in your body. Equally powerful in effect are the countless offenses you will spare your body and your beauty by leaving the old choices behind.

> **MYTH: *The well-known brands are the best.***
>
> **TRUTH: *The best products are made by companies that spend money on ingredients, not marketing.***

The cereal, hair-color, cosmetic, wholesome-snack, instant bake-mix, and diet-shake experts and the familiar names of the products they push ring in our heads, not because these products are exceptional but because of the priority placed on marketing them.

You may have been sold the idea that the most familiar, trusted brands are the best. But this is rarely the case and is, in fact, quite ironic if you look beyond the packaging to the actual substance you're buying—the part that has real impact on you and the richness of your life.

Our Social Connection with Name Brands

Name brands are part of our social fabric. As with some adults, brand identity is important to kids, who are harshly judged by the labels they wear and the foods they trade with friends from their lunch boxes. Advertising as an art form was perfected in the twentieth century, and we are still easily swayed by sophisticated ad campaigns. But making inferior choices based on unearned brand loyalty comes at great price you will only fully understand once you've made the switch to brands of true substance.

Don't be brand-loyal—be ingredient-loyal. Go for substance over packaging. Get past the smell, the bright colors, and the poetry and get down to the contents. Why reward money spent on PR and not on ingredients? Why not buy the best of the *best*, not merely the best of the mass-marketing campaigns?

If you look at the ingredients lists on two bottles of shampoo—one from a well-known beauty-products manufacturer and one from a health-conscious company—you'll realize that one company has spent all its money on packaging and marketing while the other has actually put living, biocompatible ingredients into its product.

WHAT'S INSIDE THE PACKAGE

Let's compare the ingredients of two brands of cream of mushroom soup. One is a brand your grandmother may have trusted; the other, less familiar.

Lipton Cup-a-Soup Cream of Mushroom
Ingredients: Maltodextrin, whey, partially hydrogenated soybean oil, cornstarch, salt, guar gum, mushrooms, yeast extract, lactic acid, sodium caseinate, sugar, natural flavors, onion powder, garlic powder, artificial flavor, caramel color, lactose, disodium guanylate, disodium inosinate

Imagine Foods Creamy Portobello Mushroom Soup
Ingredients: Filtered water, portobello mushrooms, organic onions, organic soy milk (filtered water, organic soybeans), mushrooms, organic

celery, organic rice flour, organic expeller-pressed safflower oil, sea salt, organic spices

Which of these do you think your body recognizes as food? Basic survival instinct demands us to know the origin of the substances we put in and on our bodies. It is counterintuitive to eat something mysterious, no matter how used to it we have become. Today you can even buy instant soups with real ingredients, so don't deprive your body in the name of convenience.

MYTH: *Synthetic products have surpassed natural ones.*

TRUTH: *Nature's sophistication is inimitable.*

We think of man-made technology as being more sophisticated, but in reality it is nature that is inimitable. Technology may help isolate, stabilize, or deliver the power of nature, but it cannot replace it. Nature works by countless mechanisms and synergies. Synthetics work by only a few, and invariably fall short in the attempt to take the place of natural substances in and on our bodies. In fact, in most cases, new problems are prone to arise. Even if the smell and the packaging have won you over, the body inevitably makes the distinction between natural and denatured.

Many plant substances, because they are bio-identical to those in the body, have the amazing ability to balance our chemistry, whether we are deficient in—or have an excess of—that substance. No synthetics can do this. For example, plant estrogens can successfully mimic and displace harmful estrogens in our bodies with weaker, beneficial estrogens, and at the same time alleviate certain symptoms of estrogen deficiency. Plant estrogens such as genistein from soy can both alleviate certain hallmarks of estrogen deficiency, such as bone loss and atherosclerosis, while actually *decreasing* breast-cancer risk associated with too much harmful estrogen—the very imbalance that often results from synthetic estrogen replacement drugs like Prempro.

Similarly, plant sterols can calm over-reactive immune responses while increasing inadequate immune response and even normalize cholesterol levels by successfully mimicking and displacing harmful cholesterol in the body without creating the imbalances or side effects associated with widely prescribed cholesterol-lowering drugs.

Another compelling observation is that in some cases natural antimicrobials such as tea tree oil have been shown to work as well or better than synthetic ones, such as the trichlosan in anti-bacterial soaps, but without creating resistant strains of bacteria as trichlosan can. Some scientists believe that natural antimicrobials are too complex for bacteria to develop resistance to.

Just as synthetics may serve some purposes in our lives without tainting or disrupting our bodies, nature isn't harmless either. There are the matters of overstimulation and imbalance, which is why "concentrated nature" such as supplements and essential oils should be used with care and supervision, particularly by pregnant women. Side effects from natural substances, however, are generally resolved upon adjusted dose or discontinued use. By the same token, because of their complexity and multipurpose nature, natural remedies that help you with one problem are also likely to have multiple good side effects.

MYTH: **If it's derived from nature, it's natural.**

TRUTH: **It's not where it comes from but what's been done with it that counts.**

Many substances derived from nature are anything *but*, and the body is perhaps the best judge of when the line between natural and refined has been crossed. Mineral oil and petroleum jelly may be derived from natural petroleum, but they are highly processed hydrocarbons that do not readily break down in the environment or on our skin. They are not only incompatible with but also block sebum while disrupting the skin's ability to regulate and receive real moisture, according to cosmetic and plant chemist Aubrey Hampton, Ph.D.

Similarly, certain natural oils can be made harmful through the process of hydrogenation, which oxidizes them. Hydrogenated fats, or "*trans*-fats," such as margarine, enter our cells and unsuccessfully stand in for healthy fats, while they confuse and disrupt anti-inflammatory, immune, and other processes in the body. Heat and solvents will deplete natural oil of vitamins, skin-beautifying sterolins, and essential fatty acids (EFAs). Even nutritional supplements can have different reactions in the body, depending on their source. The d-alpha tocopherol form of vitamin E the body uses best comes from nature, while the petro-derived synthetic version, dl-alpha tocopherol does not produce the same health benefits

In cosmetics, processing and synthesizing ingredients increases the likelihood of contamination and interaction of chemicals within a product. Carcinogenic by-products like dioxane and nitrosamines are commonly formed in highly synthetic cosmetics.

Million-dollar PR campaigns continue to tell us that synthetics are superior. They tell us that synthetics are the only way to meet demand, keep products fresh, feed the hungry, and sanitize our livestock. But food and cosmetic producers of conscience have been disproving these claims for decades and producing vastly superior products.

MYTH: *Beauty is expensive.*

TRUTH: *Keeping up the illusion of beauty is expensive.*

My beauty career has given me continual contact with some of the world's most privileged people—people who can afford just about every beauty advantage they desire: personal trainers, pilates and yoga gurus, facial peels, massages, and relaxing trips to Baja. But the truth is that the little mundane choices we make day in and day out far outweigh the impact such luxuries can have on our beauty, even if we do achieve the hard body we've just paid big bucks for. And the substances the rich put on and in their bodies more often than not match those that the rest of us put on and in our bodies, even if they come in fancier packaging or on better china.

If you find yourself worried about the money you'll spend on upgrading your food and personal-care products, consider how much you might be willing to part with for another tube of lipstick, a pair of shoes, or a manicure. Then consider how much you would be willing to pay for products that can help make you radiant for the rest of your life, not just this season. Many women would rather spend

$100 on one skirt that makes their back-side look good than pay for pure, potent body products and supplements that could actually change their shape and make strategic dressing unnecessary. They consider these expenses extravagant. But they are the real beauty splurges. They're actually much less expensive than the additional cosmetics, procedures, quick fixes, compensatory clothes, and temporary cover-ups we resort to in order to maintain the mere *illusion* of beauty.

I have consistently found that the real resistance women have to budgeting money for quality food, supplements, and skin-care products is two-fold: (1) lack of faith in their effectiveness; and (2) compartmentalizing health expenses to what is covered by insurance. This is penny-wise and future-foolish. The extra money—and perhaps the smaller shoe and lipstick collections —is a small price to pay compared to the life and vitality you forfeit by making the standard choices.

I once spent a fortune keeping up with my weight fluctuations. I never had anything to wear or enough time to apply the elaborate makeup job or achieve the perfect hair I depended on to compensate for the rest of me, which was falling apart. And the cost of the resulting medical crisis was nothing to sneeze at.

After I experienced my first real physical rewards, I came to consider each purchase as an investment in my future vitality. I learned that health was not only hope but also happiness. I also learned that health creates beauty and that once your beauty shines on its own, you don't need the expensive arsenal of clever cover-ups.

Remember: Beauty isn't expensive. Settling for "virtual vitality" while taking the real thing for granted is what will cost you untold beauty and dollars down the line.

Warning: For Some, Solutions Aren't Sexy

Some of us become so absorbed in the social and cultural allure of the virtual beauty world that the transition from novelty to solution and from distraction to clarity may threaten the very structure of our lives. The pursuits of beauty, the perfect body, and even social esteem connected with the "right" designers and the "right" products displayed on your bathroom counter can actually provide a sense of purpose, accomplishment, and social camaraderie. This never-ending cycle of trend-following leads to ceaseless "research"—generally based on ad slogans and hype—on novelty products, boastful splurges, short-term fixes, and exploitation of hopes and dollars. But you'll no longer be satisfied to merely "play" with your beauty once you truly inform yourself and taste the rewards of getting serious about it. Getting hooked in to a better world of personal-care and lifestyle options will make your new, higher beauty pursuit more rewarding and successful than any before it.

Summary

- Convenience counts. Easy access to better options fosters change.
- Demand purity, potency, proof, and appeal. You can have it all.
- Go for substance over packaging. Look beyond well-known brands.
- Get and stay hooked into the world of products and resources that support and serve you.

Use the Tools to Create Your *Self*

Beauty comes not of obligatory self-maintenance but of joyful self-creation. *You* are the only expert on yourself there can ever be. If you forfeit that role, a huge part of your potential and your truest gift to yourself and to others will be lost.

Why be content to merely survive when you can thrive with glowing, vital radiance? Aren't we each worthy of being our own passion-driven project? No one ever called a painter a fanatic for refusing to use second-rate brushes and supplies on his artwork. No one ever called a chef high-maintenance for being a stickler for freshness and quality or for demanding to know the origin of the ingredients that go into his creations. We, too, must become such passionate connoisseurs of our own unique assets.

Customize your own life and create yourself solely from the inspirations of truth, your connection with yourself, and the awe-inspiring dialogue between your body and nature's intention.

> ## *Beauty comes not of obligatory self-maintenance but of joyful self-creation.*

Applying these tools will enable you to re-attune to long-neglected needs and instincts and rebuild each area of your life, from your New Year's resolutions to your beverage choice, skin care, and your pick-me-ups, to your bathroom-cabinet staples and even your healthcare objectives. These tools will help you to build your own permanent sanctuary from bombardment, disruption, and deception. Your sanctuary will be a place in which to nurture your self-creating spirit and cultivate your glowing potential on a new foundation of the healthiest motivations and the wisest, most powerful choices.

OVERHAUL YOUR DAWN-TO-DUSK ROUTINES

We are what we repeatedly do.
Excellence then is not an act, but a habit.
—Aristotle

transformation is in the details

What we do with the most frequency and regularity—no matter how mundane—are the actions that have the greatest impact on our quality of life and our physical reflections. Too often our routines are on autopilot or by someone else's design. It's what we blindly invite into our minds, bodies, and lives that ultimately wears us down. By simply tweaking countless low-grade assaults hidden in our everyday routines, it's possible to make dozens of adjustments without feeling or missing a thing—except perhaps the chronic irritation, skin rashes, breakouts, headaches, energy leaks, and other compounded layers of short- and long-term harm we've needlessly endured.

The first step is to identify and examine our autopilot rituals, determine what isn't working, and find better options to take their place. For example, you may drink a certain beverage every day. What is the negative effect?

What if you found you liked another beverage equally well, which saved you the unhealthy effects the other had been causing and offered you immediate and cumulative beauty and health rewards? By switching to the new drink, you would shed one of many assaults your body has to recover from every day; at the same time, you would support yourself in a new way every time you drink it. In fact, the more you drank the old, beauty-sapping beverage in the past, the more dramatic and immediate the rewards of the upgrade. For example, substituting soda with a healthy spritzer (see the chart on pages 99–101) will have more tremendous skin and body payoffs for the addict than it will for people who drink soda only occasionally.

Consider your autopilot self-care habits and how you can improve upon them:

- Personal hygiene
- Beverage choices
- Skin, hair, and cosmetic regimens
- Bathroom-cabinet staples
- Food choices
- Pick-me-ups

It can take a surprisingly short amount of time—sometimes only a matter of days—for you to feel and see noticeable effects of changes made to these routines. If you make the right choices for you, it won't take long for your substitutions to become not only second nature but also your first choices. Anything that isn't agreeable within two weeks isn't the right tweak for you. And never give up if one upgrade doesn't work. There are more appealing options popping up all the time.

start linking your looks with your life

Today it is easier than ever to disconnect with our true looks because cosmetic and dermatologic technologies have allowed us to cover, sand, zap, or surgically alter ourselves. With today's sophisticated texture of makeup, skin-resurfacing techniques, and botox, we can look dewy, vibrant, and even emotionally unburdened. We often consider only the "sandability" or "zap-ability" of the flaw rather than what signs like discoloration, blemish patterns, poor circulation, or broken capillaries convey to us about our health and our choices, and we may therefore miss out on the opportunity to truly heal our beauty from the inside.

There's more to gain from looking in the mirror than assurance that our makeup is right, our teeth are clear of spinach, or our concealer is doing its job. Virgin skin—before all of the acids, peels, and irritants throw it off-kilter—is the ultimate messenger. The skin on your face changes constantly. Facial bumps, circles, and changes aren't there to embarrass us; they should alert, inspire, and guide us to take steps to correct an imbalance that is likely affecting us in countless other ways.

Doctors are increasingly less likely to give much consideration to aesthetic cues, perhaps because we've become so good at altering them superficially. How often will doctors tell you that your under-eye circles, your brittle hair and nails, your bloated abdomen, or your age spots are revealing something about your health? But any approach to health, wellness, and wholeness must be aesthetically sensitive, if not guided. If we continue to obliterate our external "flaws" without first considering the precious clues and responsive guidance they can potentially provide, we deny ourselves the rich opportunity to connect with our bodies and mirrors in a far more nurturing way.

Only *we* can attune ourselves to the revealing dialogue between our actions and our reflections. First, however, we need to slow down and quiet down to hear it. This sacred communication with our bodies is all too often disrupted by sensory bombardment, desensitizing quick fixes, drugs, chemicals, and overstimulating foods that can short-circuit our body's signals.

Once we have reached a detoxified state of healing and thriving, the naked face becomes the body's incredibly responsive messenger. It reacts to every internally or externally applied choice. As you read more of your body's messages loud and clear, occasional transient signs in the mirror lose their ability to cause panic, and the do-something impulse that leads to impatient quick fixes will be replaced with the liberating knowledge that nothing can resolve most of those signs more completely or healthily than your body once you've recovered its optimum ecology and pro-beauty functions. Some skin problems that come and go, like rashes and sensitivity, can often be phased out or greatly diminished once the dialogue between our actions and our skin has been interpreted.

establish a new relationship with your mirror

Start each morning by really looking at your face and taking in what it has to tell you. You'll begin to see marked—even startling—day-to-day fluctuations in your facial shape and features and even in your skin's tone. For example, your face can de-puff noticeably within as little as one day after weaning off refined sugar. As we become increasingly attuned to little changes in our faces and start to trace them to the offending—or healing— acts, thoughts, and substances, we begin to see flaws as more than nuisances. Each one becomes an opportunity to transform our beauty authentically from the inside out. In this way, beauty becomes a motivator that finally serves us. The so-called vanity table becomes the setting for a sacred daily ritual.

The brief, contemplative minutes at my own vanity table constitute a grounding daily check-in—a "state-of-my-beauty" address that I read from my face. I use this time to take in the astounding rewards of prior adjustments that are still paying off as well as the new changes that carry clues about more recent lifestyle shifts. Every face tells a different story, and that story can change dramatically from day to day. For example, the under-eye circles that occasionally appear in my mirror are usually from lack of sleep, the sulfites in conventional wine, or sweets. But under-eye circles can have dozens of other causes. The next time you look in the mirror, look more closely and listen carefully to how your face speaks to you about your choices and your life.

the naked experiment: deconstruct your beauty at the surface

Consider breaking unfounded beauty habits you may have started without thinking and continued for the sake of ritual or fear of stopping: the permanent wave, over-zealous brow plucking, or the trademark lipstick you just can't seem to throw out. Start from scratch. If you wear makeup or perfectly coiffed hair, try taking a break from it on weekends—as much as feels comfortable—until what feels naked at first starts to feel OK. Take note of your subtle and unique assets that may have been obscured by constructed makeup and hairstyles and allow yourself to reevaluate the effects you typically try to achieve. You may notice by going without powder, for example, that the oily condition you had been trying to control is really natural, healthy skin lubrication. You may notice the natural blush you get after you exercise and favor it over the effect you had created with makeup. Use these discoveries as inspiration for using makeup to subtly augment and even help you visualize your emerging radiance as you progress along your path to true vitality. During this period of paring down and coming to terms with the real you, use only neutral or sheer makeup colors to play up subtle contours without stealing the focus from *you*.

Most of all, free yourself of any restrictive visual persona that may have confined you in the past. If you'd always felt you *had* to wear makeup, you might want to take a break from it altogether. Then you can be sure that when you do wear it again, it really is your choice to do so. The nature of the reactions this may cause among friends and significant others will certainly reveal the rigidity and extent of the beauty prison you are escaping as well as the ability of others to focus on who you really are. Continue this external shedding by questioning every augmentation: shoulder pads, pins, scarves, loud makeup, and overly structured hair. Can you get out the door on short notice without feeling like a disaster? If not, you're not really free. But you will be. As your inner vitality unfolds, your old makeup, hair, and even wardrobe crutches will be shed naturally.

LIGHTEN UP

These strategies will get you in the spirit to break free of burdensome routines:

- **Take a break from difficult people.** If you can't, find ways to establish emotional or physical boundaries within a situation. Consider whether a bigger or more permanent change will be necessary.

- **Clear out the clutter.** Outfits should flatter even when you've got no makeup on and your hair hasn't been done. If they only work on the finished product, they don't do enough for you. Throw out clothes and accessories that may fit but don't make you feel good. You will feel your spirit lighten.

- **Get naked.** Go with less makeup or even without it, at least on weekends. Find as many things as you can to like about your naked face. As you begin to grow comfortable with it, others will too. As you continue the process of shedding and rebuilding, you may find that the bare minimum makeup—or even none at all— becomes plenty.

- **Use only the essentials.** Give up heavy synthetic perfumes. Use essential oil-based balms or skin oils. Buy olive-oil soap and naturally-scented shampoos and moisturizers.

- **Change your colors.** Break out of your regular habits. Wear white if you've been wearing only black, color if you've been wearing only neutrals, and serene or rich neutrals if you've been wearing bright colors all the time.

- **Try something new.** Start a hobby or join a class that challenges a new side of you. Make it your own secret or pursue it with a friend.

take a dawn-to-dusk self-inventory

To peel any layers of regimen buildup or problem-causing solutions you are currently burdened with, it's important to scrutinize your raw materials— what goes on and in your body, as well as your routines—and the motivation and information behind them. Here is an exercise that will provide some insight into your choices and give you baseline information about yourself. From here you can begin your shedding process.

Grab a notebook or a journal and write down your answers to these questions about your dawn-to-dusk routines. Allow a full page or more for each one. Be prepared to look at some of the products you use in order to complete this self-inventory; the more thought and specifics you put into it, the more effectively you will launch your shedding process.

Don't try to complete your own prescription of upgrades in this first exercise. You will return to this inventory to make additional notes as you read the chapters that follow, and you will solidify your own unique plan of action as you revisit your self-inventory at the end of each chapter.

Your Morning Rituals

Grooming and Beauty

- What do you see in the mirror on a typical morning before you put on your makeup? Describe the quality of your skin. Can you connect any signs on your face with the lifestyle culprit (e.g., lack of sleep or a food you ate)? Are you content with what you see? If not, what would you like to see?
- List the skin, hair, body-care products, and cosmetics you use each morning. Jot down a few words about why you chose each one.
- How do you style your hair? Do you color it? Perm it? Is it the same every day or does it vary according to your moods and what it's doing on its own? Do you have issues with the quality and texture of your hair? Do you have issues with your scalp?

Wellness and Health

- What over-the-counter medicine-cabinet staples do you reach for? List the ones you use every morning. Then list the ones you use occasionally. What are the possible side effects of each product, including those you've experienced? Can you connect any lifestyle choices with times you needed the most help from over-the-counter, symptom-controlling drugs? Have you noticed any body or skin changes since taking them?
- List the supplements you take and the benefits you seek from each one.
- List the prescription drugs you use every morning and their side effects you were either told about or have experienced firsthand. Now check the literature that comes with your prescription drugs and jot down any other side effects you haven't listed. Be aware that the side effects listed in package inserts are often incomplete or merely a list of the most apparent side effects.

Food and Drink
- List the foods and beverages you have in the morning. What do you choose on "good" days? What about "bad" days? Can you connect any beverage or food choices with how you look or feel?

Activity
- Do you fit exercise into your morning schedule? If so, what kind and how often?
- Is exercise drudgery for you or do you enjoy it? When do you like it and when do you not? Would you like to increase your activity level?
- If you smoke, when do you tend to do it? List specific times.

Environment and Mood
- How do you typically start your day? Are you focused on others? Pressed for time? Moving on autopilot? Do you look forward to the average day or are you anxious? Do you have a vice, such as eating certain foods or smoking, that is an issue in the morning?
- What goes on around you as you begin your day? Is it chaotic or quiet? Do you watch television, read the paper, listen to the radio or music, or sit quietly? Are you interrupted or left alone?

Summary
On good days I do these things:
This is what I need to work on:
This would make my mornings better:
These obstacles keep me from making those changes:
Notes and self-observations:

Your Daytime Rituals

Grooming and Beauty

- How often do you touch up your makeup and hair? Would you feel self-conscious if you couldn't touch up regularly?

Wellness and Health

- How do you feel during the day? What prescription and over-the-counter drugs do you take to get through the day? List their benefits and possible side effects.
- List any supplements you take during the day and the benefits you seek from them.

Food and Drink

- List everything you eat and drink for lunch and in the late afternoon. Include pick-me-ups and vices. Do you binge, skip meals, deprive yourself of certain foods, or need other foods? Do you need caffeine to get through the day?

Activity

- Do you get any physical activity in the normal course of your day? Is your work sedentary? Do you get fatigued or feel physical effects from your work? What adjustments could relieve those effects?
- If you smoke, drink alcohol, or binge during the day, when do you typically do it? Can you connect these habits to rituals, emotional cues, or any other triggers?

Environment and Mood

- Are you happy? Stimulated? Anxious? Utilized? Underutilized? Which parts of your day do you enjoy and which do you dislike? How is your mood at the end of a typical day? On a good day? On a bad day? Why do you feel the way you do on these days?

- What external issues set your moods and affect them during the day? Your kids? Work? Co-workers? Is your environment conducive to focus and productivity? What would improve them?
- Determine your own mood curve. For example, do you wake up in a good mood and feel anxious, tired, or depressed later? Create a graph that shows your mood as it changes throughout the day.

Summary

On good days I do these things:

This is what I need to work on:

This would make my days better:

These obstacles keep me from making those changes:

Notes and self-observations:

Your Evening Rituals

Grooming and Beauty

- What are your bedtime hygiene rituals? Write down each product and routine.

Wellness and Health

- List the drugs, health aids, and supplements you take at night and their benefits and side effects, just as you did with those you take in the morning.

Food and Drink

- List everything you eat after 5 P.M. Are you at peace with food you eat in the evening, or do you wrestle with "shoulds" and "shouldn'ts"? Do you use food for comfort? Do you binge? Do you zone out or watch television as you eat? Note which choices make you feel good and which make you feel bad. Do your food or beverage choices produce any physical discomfort, require over-the-counter digestive aids, or interfere with sleep? Can you trace how any of them affect your skin?

Activity
- Do you do any physical activity after work? If so, what do you do?
- Do you engage in any unhealthy vices after work or in the evening? If so, what are they?

Environment and Mood
- Does your evening routine set the stage for relaxing sleep, or does it leave you stressed and anxious? Do you leave behind concerns and change gears from work mode to more relaxing activities, or do you engage yourself in stressful matters before turning out the light?
- Do emotional issues dominate your evening or affect your sleep? Do you relax or feel bombarded by kids or other pressures? How are you currently dealing with these issues? Do your emotions lead to bingeing or other compulsive behaviors?

Summary
On good days I do these things:

This is what I need to work on:

This would make my evenings better:

These obstacles keep me from making those changes:

Notes and self-observations:

Self-Evaluation Questionnaire
This is your life—the mundane stuff and everything in between. Untold beauty lies dormant and untapped in the often-neglected details you are

about to address. As you review and analyze your habits and mind-sets, you can begin to visualize where there might be room for some high-dividend upgrades.

Without judging yourself, look at your self-inventory and think about the choices you make throughout the day. Try to grasp their cumulative effects. Each choice has an impact on the larger story of your life.

The following questionnaire is intended to prime your thoughts in preparation for the active steps in the chapters to come.

- What "fixes" get you through the day? Which activities or products help you thrive?
- Hair and makeup aside, what could the mirror be telling you? Have you been healing and thriving or merely reacting and surviving?
- Identify your most frequent autopilot routines. Are there products you use every day that you haven't scrutinized? Do you eat or apply anything without knowing what's in it?
- Are your routines and choices informed, or have you left some details to chance? How are your choices informed? Are they influenced by social or marketing cues, cravings, dependencies, popular trends, or convenience?
- Look at your personal-care choices. Could any of your skin or health regimens be causing new problems or irritation?
- Look at your drugs and bathroom-cabinet quick fixes. Have you been covering a growing problem or a coming crisis?
- Now focus on your foods and beverages. Do you see a pattern between your choices and how you feel and look?
- What are your current beauty worries and priorities?
- What are your current beauty splurges, and what priorities, preferences, and information are they based on?
- How do you approach your skin and body issues? Do you have a comprehensive get-to-the-cause attitude or a surface sand-and-zap attitude?

- How much do budget and convenience affect your choices?
- Do you prefer certain brand-name products? Why?
- Do beautiful packaging and poetic passages on the label make you overlook ingredients listed in small print?
- Are you satisfied with products that appear natural even if you're not really sure they are?
- Are any of your choices impulsive or compulsive?
- Are any of your habits perpetuated by emotional triggers or cravings?

re-sensitize your senses by detoxifying your rituals

It is surprisingly easy to work around the beauty wild cards of regimen overkill, food additives, and chemicals that muffle or distort our bodies' messages. By minimizing this disruptive "noise" choice by choice, we can re-attune ourselves to the sacred dialogue between nature and our bodies and learn to follow our body's lead again.

As you begin detoxifying your regimens and rituals, you may notice your body becoming more sensitive. It's not that your body is less tolerant; rather, it is improving its communication. As a result, you'll preserve your precious vitality by uncovering crises *before* they happen.

shed the three types of beauty self-sabotage

There are three types of self-sabotage that are important to target in your process of shedding:

- *Unwitting self-sabotage.* These are choices we haven't scrutinized or have adopted based on incomplete information. These products can easily be weeded out with good information and simple upgrades.
- *Assisted self-sabotage.* This is when we let ourselves be led by fads, dubious diet and beauty trends, industry agendas, or convenience

issues at our own expense. Good information and products, the proper motivation, and some practical logistical strategies should nip this kind of self-sabotage in the bud.

- *Compulsive self-sabotage.* These are addictive vices such as smoking, overeating, or drinking. Compulsive self-sabotage is tougher to kick because you not only have the issues associated with the other types of self-sabotage but also the emotional and chemical issues on top of them, all feeding and perpetuating each other. If you have a vice you want to correct, there's nothing wrong with setting a quitting date, but understand that the more contributing factors you shed in the meantime, the greater your odds of quitting, the less your struggle, and the more real your success will be.

Certain chemical conundrums that affect your body may have a direct impact on your success in letting go of unhealthy habits and behaviors. They include

- Nutritional deficiencies, food sensitivities, and blood-sugar issues
- Mood-affecting chemical imbalances, such as low serotonin levels
- Hormonal imbalances that affect weight and appetite
- Skin imbalances caused by sensitizing products
- Over-the-counter and prescription drug side effects
- Environmental and household toxins that challenge the body

Correcting or minimizing these issues is not only possible but also a crucial factor is the process of shedding. Quitting a negative habit or vice cold turkey only works if the person has already shed the key factors supporting it and is thus primed for the final, successful attempt. The process of shedding brings these issues to the surface, reconnects us with our inner dialogue, feeds our sense of self-respect, and alleviates the toxic burdens and the depletion that are too often stacked against us.

THINGS TO DO TO HONOR YOUR TRUE BEAUTY

The following tips from the IDentity Project constitute an uplifting checklist for breaking with self-destructive mind-sets and self-talk.

1. Start each morning by looking in the mirror and saying something self-affirming about yourself out loud.

2. Consciously choose to avoid making comments about other people or yourself based on the way they look, such as "You look so skinny," which is an objectification of the recipient of your comments, or "I need to lose weight," which is defaming to yourself.

3. Compliment other people for skills, talents, or characteristics they have that you appreciate.

4. Enjoy the whole, real food that you love without shame, and experience nourishing your body without counting anything.

5. Throw out all of your "diet" foods and products and your bathroom scale.

6. Don't read magazines that promote negative feelings about weight, body image, and food. Instead, read a book that lifts your self-esteem, promotes positive body image, encourages healthy living, or helps you overcome stereotypes about social standards of beauty.

7. Find time for stillness away from television, advertisements, and popular culture.

8. Focus on creative pursuits and self-enrichment.

make your doctor a part of the process

Part of the process of shedding involves working with your doctor to uncover unresolved health issues. Shift your mind-set from covering the symptom to getting to the cause. Allergies, yeast infections, headaches, and cold hands and feet all provide clues to other issues that, if left unresolved, can steal your beauty and quality of life, even if you are living a pro-beauty lifestyle. The next time you take another antacid or aspirin or apply another steroid cream, be sure to revisit any symptom you've been muffling and give it your full consideration. Problems and any symptoms should be pursued until causes are ruled out one by one. If your doctor won't take interest in getting to the bottom of your body and skin complaints, then consider finding another who will. Later on we'll explore several ways to make your time with your doctor part of your higher objective toward true health and radiance.

In the meantime, keep your self-inventory with this book. Jot down the pro-beauty lifestyle upgrades, strategies, and products you'd like to try as you read each chapter and as you study the Living Beauty Resource Guide. If you focus on your most frequent autopilot routines, your first cycle of upgrades will give you enough short- and long-term rewards to inspire and propel you into your next cycle of upgrades. You'll notice that there is always a shedding aspect to any new act as you leave each beauty assault behind. This is the key to the process of shedding—not deprivation but informed, uplifting choices that lighten your beauty burdens one by one and make you feel better in your spirit and in the flesh each time you apply them.

With inspiration from the following chapters, the Resources, and the tangible physical rewards you have coming, you'll be hooked to an ever-expanding world of exciting and liberating ways to look and live better. Let's get started!

Part II

FEEDING AND CULTIVATING BEAUTY

Chapter 5

DRINK YOURSELF BEAUTIFUL

It's easy to become mindful of what we eat while tuning out how we quench our thirst. Because of the consistency, frequency, and sheer volume of our drink choices, habitual sips, slurps, and gulps can have more impact on our looks and well-being than just about anything else we do. Virtually every beauty factor—skin, hair, bones, weight, breast health, and overall vitality—is dramatically affected by the beverages we drink every day. Whether that effect is positive or negative is up to us. Fortunately, our drink habits are incredibly easy to tweak for astounding immediate and cumulative beauty rewards.

You may already be the proud owner of an evolved palate and enjoy beauty-enhancing beverages like pure water, green tea, herbal concoctions, and even creamy or sweet drinks with minimal sugar and caffeine. If that is the case, this chapter will provide you with added motivation, an expanded repertoire of exciting new pro-beauty beverage tastes, and increased physical rewards. But if you are a regular drinker of beauty-stealing beverages such as sweetened commercial teas, sodas, fruit drinks, iced-coffee concoctions, or even juice and are apprehensive about giving them up, you stand to reap the most dramatic immediate rewards if you change what you drink. Your face may respond to a well-chosen upgrade with reduced puffiness and under-eye circles as soon as tomorrow morning. If you are currently a slave to your fifteen-dollar-a-week mochalattechococcino habit, you may enjoy clearer, smoother skin in as little as two weeks simply by upgrading to truly hydrating brews in lieu of dehydrators like coffee.

this is not about calories

As kids we learn that sugar rots our teeth. As grown-ups we learn that sugar drives up the *calorie* content of what we eat and drink. We also learn that coffee speeds up our metabolism so we can burn more *calories* and that sugar-free drinks won't affect our diets because they contain no *calories*. But the calories we tally are not the real problem; it's the unstable chemistry of cravings, energy, and moods that sugary, caffeinated, and diet drinks can perpetuate. As you continue with your series of upgrades, you'll see that it is the healing, balancing, and truly satiating qualities in drinks and foods that matter most to your looks and your life in the long and even the short run.

We make jokes all the time about our sugar and caffeine addictions without really considering the truth behind our words. These addictions have real physiological effects on our bodies. The secret to breaking this cycle is the simple act of upgrading—not sacrificing.

strategic upgrades and taste-bud training

Your initial goal should be to find satisfying and revitalizing upgrades for any beauty-robbing beverages you drink. This will have quick physical payoffs and free you of the chemical pendulum that can cause you need-less cravings and energy slumps. Upgrading your beverage also changes how you taste foods, which is why this chapter is the crucial strategic jump-start to the series of food upgrades that follow in the next chapter.

Well-chosen substitutions that are right for you won't feel like substitu-tions at all after the first few days. This sometimes requires a little experi-mentation, but when you find the right ones, rather than feeling deprived, all you will feel are the old burdens lifting away, the new beauty effects set-ting in, and new taste sensations pleasing your palate. You'll wonder how you ever did without your new choices.

start with pure water: the least and the most you can do for your beauty

At least 70 percent of the skin's blemish- and wrinkle-fighting hydration comes from the water we consume. If I've just motivated you to drink more water—good! Just be sure you're not drinking more *tap* water. If you haven't done so already, switching from chlorinated tap water—the water you shower in—to reliably purified water will be perhaps the most important health and beauty lifestyle upgrade you will ever make. If you do not have a water purifier, then I would wager that you are not much of a water drinker. It's hard to make yourself drink a healthy quantity of water if it tastes bad, and it is unhealthy to drink a lot of heavy metals, volatile organic chemicals, and chlorine—which ages the body and skin and impedes the body's ecology.

Here are some motivations to upgrade to pure water:

- Clearer, more comfortable skin as body ecology is re-established
- A slowdown of your aging process
- A healthier digestive tract and better absorption of nutrients.
- Diminished allergies and yeast infections with improved bacterial balance

Pure water will boost the value and appeal of every tea, soup, and beverage you make at home. See the Resources for some of the best water purifiers and distillers for the money as well as the first pitcher-type and portable purifiers that work well and are affordable. Water purifiers are the best beauty bang for the buck!

IS INSULIN RESISTANCE WEIGHING YOU DOWN?

Insulin normalizes blood-sugar levels in the body. Insulin resistance, which affects nearly fifty million Americans, is a condition in which a body's cells build up tolerance to insulin, which makes the body less effective at doing its job of keeping blood sugar stable. Feeling tired after eating and being overweight are common symptoms of insulin resistance. Sometimes called "Syndrome X" or "metabolic syndrome," it can lead to more serious problems such as diabetes and heart disease. Foods and beverages high in refined sugars contribute to insulin resistance by causing a spike in blood-sugar levels. Humans are not built to handle that much sugar, and we don't show any sign of adapting to it. Fortunately, this condition can be prevented, greatly improved, or even reversed by avoiding sugar, eating more fiber, being active, and stopping smoking, all of which make the cells more sensitive to insulin. Luckily, there's a sweet yet healthy upgrade for every liquid sugar fix you crave.

sweet drinks are even worse than sweet foods

If you're sensitive to sugar like most people, a jolt of sugar such as your morning juice will start a pendulum of mood swings and cravings that will continue throughout the day. Liquid sugar does crazy things to the body. In addition to causing the pancreas to spew too much insulin in order to neutralize the massive sugar rush, it also causes the excess sugar (or carbohydrates) to be stored as fat. In this way, sugar can actually turn our bodies into fat-storing machines, even if we're not eating any fat. The concentrated nature of beverages allows sugar to enter the bloodstream more quickly, so sugary drinks are often even more likely than food to cause fat gain. Eating an orange, however, introduces sugar into the bloodstream slowly because of the fiber that fruit has, but drinking orange juice is more like mainlining sugar. It's easy to become addicted to liquid sugar's immediate lift while becoming a victim of its unwanted consequences, but it's avoidable if you strategize some palate-pleasing upgrades.

SWEET CHOICES

Stevia

Stevia is an herb three hundred times sweeter than sugar. It can't be patented in its naturally occurring form, which is why you may not have heard about it.

Stevia has been used as a sweetener in Japan for decades and in South America for centuries. Indigenous tribes in Brazil actually used stevia to treat diabetes, and today some studies have demonstrated that it can stabilize blood sugar. The FDA has not approved stevia as a food additive, and therefore it cannot be promoted as a sweetener; however, you can buy it at health-food stores in convenient packets. You can also buy the plant or the seed to grow your own.

SlimSweet® and Lo Han Sweet™

If SlimSweet is what it appears to be, we may have a perfect no-calorie, no-chemical sweetener in our midst. It's a very tasty—but very expensive—and apparently natural sweetener that has recently appeared on the market. SlimSweet is made from a "blend" called Lo Han Gold,® and the Glycemic Research Institute has determined it to be low-glycemic and safe for most diabetics. Another natural sweetener, called Lo Han Sweet,™ made with Lo Han and xylitol, just hit the market and is the best one yet in my opinion. Still low in calories and glycemic index, it is actually good for the teeth. Both SlimSweet™ and Lo Han Sweet™ work well in cooking. See the Resources.

Splenda®

The great-tasting, though synthetic, Splenda (sucralose) was approved by the FDA in 1998. Much of it cannot be absorbed by the digestive tract, and it has not produced tumors in lab studies as some other artificial sweeteners have. For this reason, many people are comfortable using it. Note that FDA findings regarding the animal tests on Splenda show thymus gland shrinkage and kidney swelling when Splenda was administered in very high quantities. Splenda merits more independent, long-term investigation, as any synthetic chemical does. I consume the occasional Splenda-sweetened item, but I am more comfortable with stevia, Slim-Sweet, or Lo Han Sweet in my drinks and recipes.

sugar and skin

In his book *The Perricone Prescription* (HarperCollins, 2002), Nicholas Perricone, M.D., points out the compelling scientific connections between sugar and everything from inflammation, blemishes and edema-related puffiness, and under-eye circles to wrinkles, sagging, brown spots, and overall accelerated aging. He explains how sugar can also wreak havoc on collagen, leading to the cross-linking of the fibers that give elasticity to the skin, thereby causing wrinkles. In addition, it is now known that another aging process caused by sugar, called glycation, results in an ugly type of protein breakdown in the skin and throughout the body.

If you regularly consume beverages with upwards of 18 grams of sugar per serving—the same as a Hershey bar and less than in a glass of grapefruit juice—you not only have serious motivation to make the substitutions suggested in the following chart but also incredible beauty rewards to look forward to.

Here are some motivations to upgrade your sugar fix:
- A slimmer, sleeker body
- A dramatically refined facial appearance due to diminished puffiness
- Smoother, clearer skin—and fewer wrinkles in your future
- Better skin color with reduced sensitivity
- Elimination of a primary cause of premature aging
- Victory over cravings

Gradually decreasing consumption of beverages high in sugar will naturally help you to painlessly do the same in the food upgrades that follow your Beverage Makeover. Try using a healthy sweetener instead of sugar. After only a two- or three-day break from the old sugar assaults, your cravings for sugar will diminish, and you will begin to taste the unique flavors in real drinks with much greater interest and appreciation.

get the support you need to wean off sugar
Though the body's call for nourishment is seemingly silenced by a sugar fix, many people don't realize that nutritional deficiencies can actually be *caused*

FRUIT SPRITZERS:
THE PERFECT SODA UPGRADE

Fruit spritzers quench thirst on a whole new level. They are so easy to make that you can do them at home or even order them at your favorite restaurant or bar. You can start with one-quarter juice and reduce it as your tastebuds adjust.

Basic Recipe
Plain soda water with a splash of orange, apple, grapefruit, or grape juice and a twist of lime

Kat's Favorite Cranberry and Pomegranate Spritzers
Follow the basic recipe, but instead of the juices listed, add a splash of unsweetened cranberry or pomegranate juice for a beautiful blush (see Resources for availability). Since pomegranate is naturally sweet and cranberry is tart, the combination is refreshing. A pinch of stevia powder will bring out the sweetness. This is a real soda substitute that satisfies the sweet, fizzy, and soda cravings all at once. And there are added bonuses: Cranberry juice can clear up and prevent bladder infections, and pomegranate juice contains healthy phyto-estrogens and has proven benefits to the heart. Both are high in vitamin C. On top of all that, they're delicious!

by sugar. These deficiencies are widespread—even for those who eat a balanced diet. With the support of the beverage and food upgrades to come and the blood-sugar-stabilizing supplements you'll read about in chapter 8, your body's needs will be met in a way that satisfies its deepest hunger and thirst, and it will remain satisfied until true hunger—not just craving—strikes.

diet drinks don't work and may be dangerous

Scientific studies have not shown any long-term weight loss or prevention of weight gain from consumption of artificially sweetened diet drinks. In fact, beyond the bone-destructive phosphates in diet sodas, there may be some serious dangers lurking in all aspartame-sweetened diet drinks.

According to nutritional pioneer Dr. Michael B. Schachter, co-author of *Food, Mind and Mood*, 80 to 85 percent of all complaints received by the FDA are attributed to aspartame. Between 1984, when the FDA approved aspartame, and 1987, the FDA had received more than six thousand complaints concerning aspartame, including 250 involving epileptic seizures. Dr. Shachter explains: "If an approved drug had as many complaints as aspartame, it probably would have been removed from the market long ago. But, aspartame has been approved as a food additive, not a drug, so the manufacturer doesn't have to track adverse reactions as they would with a drug.

"Aspartame, like MSG, is an 'excitotoxin,'" Dr. Schachter further explains. "Because its effects are cumulative, one may feel fine consuming it at first, then begin to experience problems characteristic of the headache, vision, and other neurological complaints regularly called in. An additional concern about aspartame is that it tends to lower serotonin in the brain. Low brain serotonin levels are associated with depression."

The FDA responds to concerns about aspartame by saying that methanol (a potentially harmful by-product of aspartame) is common in fruits and vegetables. But several prominent scientists, including Dr. Schachter, board-certified neurosurgeon Dr. Russell L. Blaylock, and Dr. H. J. Roberts, author of *Aspartame (Nutrasweet): Is It Safe?* note that while natural methanol in fruits is commonly offset by the presence of ethanol, the methanol in aspartame is without protective ethanol, so it can be absorbed and may cause harm as it accumulates.

Acesulfame K and Saccharin

Acesulfame K (Sunette®), also listed as acesulfame potassium, has increasingly been used in protein shakes and other beverages since 1988 and, like saccharin, has been linked with tumor growth in animal studies.

Fortunately, you now know about the safer alternatives, so you needn't become another lab rat.

Here are some motivations to upgrade your diet drinks:

- Fewer cravings and less overeating caused by seratonin-lowering aspartame
- Stronger bones if you upgrade from sodas, which contain bone-eating phosphates
- Peace of mind and freedom from the possible consequences of aspartame

Consider the upgrades I suggest in the "Beverage Makeovers" chart (pages 99–101) for diet drinks. Try using one of the alternative sweeteners in the "Sweet Choices" sidebar (pages 81–82) for teas, coffee or coffee substitutes, spritzers, and lemonade—and also in foods. The upgrades I suggest for diet drinks are the same you would choose for sugary beverages. And don't be concerned if the upgrade contains more calories. As you will learn in the next chapter, not all calories are equal, and it's likely that drinking more calories in the form of low-sugar upgrades from the "Beverage Makeovers" chart will result in healthy weight loss.

caffeine, cravings, and fatigue

Dr. Schachter explained the caffeine-fatigue connection to me: "Coffee and other caffeine sources cause the release of stress ('fight or flight') hormones, which has two negative effects. The first is a blood-sugar drop, followed by increased sugar cravings; the second is increased fatigue over time that is caused by the exhaustion of the adrenal glands, which

RESTORE YOUR PRO-BEAUTY ALKALINE BALANCE

One of the surest steps to better skin and vitality is to alkalize your body, according to Dr. Susan Lark, editor of *The Lark Letter* and co-author of *The Chemistry of Success*:

"Most of the chemical processes within the body work optimally in an alkaline pH of 7.3 to 7.4. The dead giveaway that you're acidic is low bone density or osteoporosis, in which the bones are thin and porous. The bones will leech their minerals into the blood to maintain the body's slightly alkaline state. Women with big, strong bones are more alkaline and do best on a meat-based diet with lots of fruits and vegetables while overly acidic women with low bone density do well with a mineral-rich diet that emphasizes vegetables, legumes, and grains."

The ideal pH level is 7.0 or slightly higher. You can buy pH-testing strips from most pharmacies and test the pH of your saliva or urine.

inevitably occurs in those who consume caffeine throughout the day over extended periods. The result is burnout and fatigue."

Caffeine can also cause insulin resistance. Furthermore, caffeine can contribute to elevated cortisol, a stress hormone, according to Stephen Cherniske,

Acidifying Beverages	Alkalizing Beverages
• Sugary drinks	• Lemon water
• Milk	• Kefir
• Coffee	• Teeccino (see sidebar on page 89)

M.S., author of *Caffeine Blues*. In this book, he describes how this condition affects sleep and causes immunity problems, accelerated aging, and mood changes. Cortisol has also been linked to accumulation of abdominal fat. As cortisol rises, the body's level of DHEA—the "youth hormone"—decreases. That's bad news for your beauty and quality of life.

Here are some motivations to upgrade your caffeine fix:

- Freedom from cravings caused by coffee's blood–sugar connection
- Clearer, healthier skin due to increased hydration and restored alkalinity in the body
- Recovery of adrenal glands, which leads to more energy and less reactive skin
- Diminished under-eye puffiness as cortisol-related water retention is reduced
- Stronger bones because of increased mineral absorption and better digestion
- Deeper sleep, and thus more beautifying human growth hormone (hGH) secretion during sleep
- Easier weight loss, a flatter abdomen, and slower aging from raised DHEA and lowered cortisol levels

weaning off sugar and caffeine

All sugar and caffeine fixes are related to and affected by each other. If you focus only on omitting your afternoon sugar fix and continue your morning juice habit, for example, you are overlooking a huge contributor to your daylong cravings and thwarting your own progress toward freedom from them. It is much easier to gradually upgrade by consistently reducing caffeine and sugar content in each beverage throughout the day. For example, if you normally drink a sweet beverage in the morning and another in the afternoon and each contain more than 20 grams of sugar, try upgrading both to beverages with only 15 grams of sugar each.

STELLAR COFFEE UPGRADE: TASTING IS BELIEVING

Teeccino is a beverage that does the impossible. It tastes, smells, and brews almost exactly like coffee in your machine, drip cone, or French press. Even die-hard coffee drinkers will be impressed. It actually restores energy (via potassium), alkaline balance, hydration, and mineral reserves rather than draining them like coffee. You can find it at your health-food store.

I brew it strong in my coffeemaker with lots of steamed milk or organic half-and-half. It is also great iced. Sweeten, if you'd like, with a dusting of one of my recommended alternative sweeteners.

Like any other vice, the allure of addictive beverages is connected to the sensory experience, chemical effects, ritual, and situation. Don't ignore your very real needs by attempting to become your own drill sergeant. Deciding to quit coffee today without considering those needs will only limit your success. Instead of focusing on self-denial, focus on satisfying each area of need your coffee fulfills.

three coffee-weaning techniques

1. More milk, less coffee. To start? Latte over cappuccino. Ask for only one espresso shot when you order the large size. Better yet, order regular coffee but ask them to fill it only halfway and top it off with milk or, as a treat, steamed milk. Over time, increase the milk to three-quarters. (Stop worrying about fat calories—just skip the sugar!) Use low-fat milk if it makes you feel better, but letting go of the fat phobia will give you a more savory, truly satisfying beverage. If you have trouble digesting milk, you might experiment with plain soy milk, which is now available at many coffeehouses. (See the soy-milk sidebar on page 96 for the best choices.)

2. Mix brews. Start mixing Teeccino in with the coffee grounds you brew at home. Gradually increase the portion of Teechino until you are drinking very little or no coffee at all.

3. Half-caf. Drink coffee that's a combination of regular and decaffeinated coffee. Keep in mind that even with decaf, you are still left with several issues that work against beauty, such as acidosis and malabsorption. Use this technique as a last resort and choose Swiss water process decaf whenever possible since other decafs generally contain toxic solvent residues like hexane.

make tea your healthy new addiction

These easy-to-love teas can intrigue your taste buds and become your new healthy addictions. *Camellia sinensis,* the only plant leaf correctly called "tea," gives us black, green, oolong, and white teas. It has taken science by storm with its proven antioxidant, anti-inflammatory, and anticancer benefits. The more tea you drink, the more beautiful and healthy your skin and body will be. Habitual tea drinking has been proven to help preserve bone density and is linked with greatly reducing the risk of heart attack. Following are some of the tastiest teas. You can drink them hot or iced. Sweeten them with a sugar alternative if you'd like, although you may eventually prefer, as I do, to fully experience them without sugar. Add milk, cream, or soy milk to scratch that cozy, creamy, dessert-and-coffee itch. And with the organic decaffeinated versions of many teas, your dreams will be sweeter, too.

Chai (Minus the Sugar)

Everything in unsweetened chai is great for you. The black tea, turmeric, and clove all have rejuvenating effects. The problem lies in the sugar that manufacturers and coffeehouses add so you will stay addicted to it. At the coffeehouse, ask them to use a chai tea bag instead of their prepared version. Leave enough room for plenty of milk. (For a creamy treat, request steamed organic milk or soy milk.) If you need it sweeter, use healthy sweetener from packets you can carry in your purse.

BETTER BOTTLED DRINKS AND TEAS

These truly refreshing bottled drinks won't spike your blood sugar, and they are convenient upgrades from sweeter bottled iced teas, juices, and other sugary drinks. Choose one that gently allows your taste buds to evolve. For example, if you're weaning off heavy-duty, sweetened iced teas, you may need to work your way down the sugar gram scale from the 24 grams found in most bottled drinks to 11 and then to 5.

Sugar content in grams:
- Ito En Teas: 0 g
- Honest Teas: 0–9 g
- Tazo Enlightened Lemon: 8 g
- V-8 juice: 11 g

Black Tea

An easy full- or part-time substitute for hot or iced coffee with antioxidant benefits similar to—though less powerful—than those of green or white tea is black tea. It contains about half the caffeine of coffee. To the evolved palate, unsweetened iced tea is divine!

Earl Grey Tea and Earl Grey Green Tea

The bergamot oil that gives Earl Grey its distinctive taste is heaven. Earl Grey is fantastic with a little organic half-and-half and is incredible iced. If you like to drink tea later in the day or if you don't react well to any amount of caffeine, I recommend an organic decaf, such as Choice or Yogi Tea brands.

Cocoa Spice Tea

Cocoa Spice Tea, from Yogi Tea, is made from cocoa beans and spices and fills the cozy, creamy, and chocolate need. It's a viable substitute for hot cocoa—which is essentially chocolate-flavored sugar-water, unless you make your own with real chocolate and an alternative sweetener. Cocoa Spice Tea is great with hot milk or soy milk, with or without sweetener.

Green Tea: The All-Star Beauty Beverage

A great place to start—and maybe even end—your search for the perfect beauty brew is green tea, which arguably contains the most benefits of any drink. Green tea has proven anti-inflammatory benefits to the skin, strengthens the teeth, decreases insulin resistance, inhibits breast cancer, burns fat, and is good for the heart. The list goes on and on. Studies have shown decreased breast-cancer risk in Japanese women proportionate to how many cups of green tea they drink per day. Among those who drank

L-THEANINE: THE FEEL-GOOD CHEMICAL IN GREEN TEA

The caffeine in green tea can be anywhere from negligible to as much as half that in coffee, but the effects of the caffeine are thought to be countered by the presence of a calming amino acid called L-theanine, which is found in decaffeinated green tea. The Japanese, who are always ahead in the health game, have been putting this natural upper in all sorts of foods and supplements for years.

the most cups in a day (six to ten small cups) were the fewest occurrences of breast cancer.

The Benefits Are Worth Acquiring a Taste For

Most green teas taste grassier than black tea, which is fermented and contains fewer antioxidants. Some people like mint, lemongrass, or other herbs in combination with green tea, and your health-food store carries plenty of these concoctions. Be wary of bottled green teas at the supermarket—no matter how clever or Zen-like the packaging—unless the sugar content is around 5 grams or less. Also avoid cheaper decaffeinated green teas that have not been decaffeinated by the carbon-dioxide method since they may have lost their beneficial properties in the decaffeination process. White tea (which is the same leaf as green) may have the most benefits of all.

Exotic Green Teas: A Connoisseur's Beauty Splurge

Creamy Taiwanese oolong, Earl Grey green, fresh jasmine tea: these are all green teas, but they taste very different from basic green tea. (Taiwanese

MY GLASS-JAR TRICK

Today I brew green teas and herbal infusions almost every day. I fill a half-gallon, heat-proof mason jar with boiling purified water, drop in a large tea ball full of tea leaves, and brew as recommended by the supplier. Sometimes I pour the water over loose jasmine pearls and watch the leaves unfold gracefully. I drink tea hot or iced every day. I choose my brew based on the kind of support my body needs that day or that week. To familiarize yourself with the beauty and body benefits of various teas, see the "Drinkable Herbs" chart on page 102.

oolong is actually buttery, and drinking jasmine tea is like drinking flowers.) It is hard to believe that something so delicious can act so powerfully on behalf of our beauty and wellness, but only a liter of oolong tea daily helped reduce allergy-related dermatitis lesions in Japanese test subjects over a few weeks. Almost all teas are great iced. Once you find one you love, you've settled on one of the ultimate pro-beauty upgrades. Mail-order sources for these and some other high-end teas and herbal infusions are listed in the Resources.

drinking for detox

Drinking pure water and every other beverage upgrade I've suggested will help detoxify your body, but if you really want a detox "event" that perks up both body and skin, go for freshly extracted dark green vegetable juices. They are alkalizing and rich in healing enzymes and chlorophyll, which has been shown in studies to carry heavy-metal pollutants out of the body. Unlike fruit juices, green vegetable juices generally won't throw off your blood sugar or make you store fat and are therefore truly energizing and nutrient-dense upgrades. (Carrot and beet juices can be combined with green juices if the taste is too strong for you, or try adding an inch of ginger root and the juice of half a lemon to make even the most potent combinations quite palatable.) If juicing is impractical, find a juice bar or health-food store that will make the juice you want, or use powdered "green drinks" that you can mix with water or make into smoothies (see the Resources).

the best liquid bone builders

In early 2002, the eye-opening results of Harvard's famous Nurse's Health Study of over seventy-seven thousand women, published in the *American Journal of Epidemiology*, showed no decrease in osteoporosis in women who drank three glasses of milk a day over those who drank none. Studies have shown that our levels of vitamin K (found in dark, leafy greens) influence

KAT'S BEAUTY DETOX ELIXIR

You can make this at home if you have a juicer, or you can have it prepared at a health-food store. I find it helps to give this list of ingredients to the person doing the juicing for easier ordering.

 1 3-inch wedge of cabbage

 1/2 large beet

 A couple bunches of dark greens (parsley, spinach, kale, or
  watercress)

 1 large carrot

 1 unpeeled lemon

 A thumb-sized piece of ginger root

Scrub—don't peel—your produce. Then cut everything up and run it all through a juicer. The benefits of this drink are out of this world: Cabbage heals the stomach lining. Beet is a terrific blood cleanser and wonderful for the skin. Dark greens are the ultimate detoxifiers and bone builders. Carrots are loaded with skin-, vision-, and body-healing carotenoids. Lemon alkalizes the body, and the peel is loaded with bioflavonoids. Ginger improves circulation and digestion.

whether the calcium we take in winds up in our bones or in our arteries. This is another reason to drink green vegetable juices whenever you can.

soy milk

Do your bones a favor and consider drinking and using soy milk instead of milk. The protein in soy has been associated with decreased risk of developing osteoporosis. It can be substituted for virtually any milk drink and can be enjoyed alone or in cold cereal, oatmeal, Teeccino, or as a dessert beverage. Heated, it's lovely on its own or in tea. The isoflavones in soy have been shown to prevent breast tumors in animal studies. But before you go overboard on soy or soy supplements, be aware that there is a bit of controversy regarding soy (see chapter 13). I also encourage you to experiment with rice, oat, and almond milks, which can be found in health-food stores. Each of these options has its own distinct taste and benefits. Remember to keep the sugar content around 11 grams or fewer.

CHOOSE YOUR BEST SOY MILK

Just visit the soy-milk section at the health-food store and you'll see the wide array of brands to choose from. If you are looking for soy milk to go with your cereal, try Silk, which tastes very much like milk because it's not too sweet. Westsoy makes the only unsweetened vanilla soy milk, which is brilliant since the maple flavoring creates a sweet "illusion."

Sugar grams in soy milk:
Westsoy Unsweetened Vanilla: 0g
Edensoy Unsweetened: 0g
Silk (Plain): 4g
Edensoy Extra (plain): 7g
Pacific Ultra (plain): 10g
Edensoy Vanilla: 15g

enjoy milk if it agrees with you

The only reason to dislike dairy (unless you're lactose-intolerant or vegan) is the tainting of cows and their milk with hormones and pesticides in recent decades. Since pesticides accumulate in the fat of conventionally raised animals, going for organic dairy products may be more important than buying organic fruits and vegetables. Even in the case of soy and other milks, buying organic saves you from being the guinea pig for genetically modified ingredients—often the soy itself, unless it's organic—and other unsavories.

If you have no problem digesting dairy products, then I encourage you to enjoy lattes and chai. Cultured dairy products like natural yogurt, buttermilk, and kefir (a yogurt drink) are far easier to digest than milk and are better for you because their active "good" bacteria cultures actually digest the lactose, improving your digestion. They're also great for the skin.

the truth about alcohol

According to the largest study on alcohol and breast cancer, published in February 1998 in the *Journal of the American Medical Association*, the alcohol equivalent of two to four shots of hard liquor per day increases breast-cancer risk by 41 percent. Similarly, a recent analysis of fifty-three epidemiological studies found that a woman's risk of breast cancer increased by 7 percent for each alcoholic drink consumed per day. Alcohol also interferes with deep-wave sleep, the type of sleep during which hGH—which heals and rejuvenates the body and skin—is released. The preservatives in wine and beer, which include sulfites, can give many people that puffy "hangover" face, under-eye circles, and headaches.

Drinking red wine moderately to protect against heart disease may be a viable upgrade from other types of alcohol, but don't delude yourself into thinking that it is better to drink than not to drink. Resveratrol supplements provide one of the key phytochemicals believed to be responsible for the heart protection that red wine offers without the known hazards of alcohol consumption.

If you are battling an alcohol addiction, be sure to seek an addiction program through your local hospital or the organizations listed in the

Resources. If you drink moderately but regularly, the blood sugar–stabilizing and liver-protecting supplements in chapter 8 may help you minimize the consequences.

target specific beauty rewards with drinkable herbs

Your initial substitutions for coffee and sugary drinks might have the most significant effects of any beverage upgrades on your beauty. But why stop there? With a more refined palate and a growing appreciation for a wider range of tastes, you can promote your beverages to "beauty elixir" status. By targeting your specific concerns, you can quench an even deeper body thirst while improving concerns such as rashes, fever blisters, bones, hair, nails, teeth, breast health, varicose veins, and even your libido. In order to gain a therapeutic effect from infusions and teas, you generally need to drink several cups throughout the day, so it's important to begin by identifying the tastes you truly enjoy.

lose the sugar in your shakes and smoothies

The terms "protein shake" and "smoothie" always sound like a healthy snack or breakfast choice, and when made right, they can give you the stable energy and nutrients you need. But they can also invite a lot of rationalization when it comes to the super-sweet concoctions some people call healthy.

The best way to upgrade the shake you like is to minimize the sugar content (skip the juice) and upgrade the quality of both the protein (cross-filtered, ion-exchange whey protein is the form the body absorbs easily) and the fruits (upgrade from bananas to berries, for starters). (Be sure to steer clear of acesulfame K–sweetened drinks.) You'll learn about the healthiest fruit choices in the next chapter.

your beverage makeover

Following is a quick reference guide to help you find a pro-beauty beverage upgrade for each beauty-robbing choice you may be drinking. You'll also

Your Beverage Makeovers

UPGRADE YOUR	FROM	TO	BEAUTY INCENTIVES
Caffeine Fix	• Coffee • Caffeinated sodas • Caffeinated teas, including commercial iced teas (see also Sugar Fix upgrades)	• Teeccino • Tea *Energy Alternatives:* • "Green" drinks, such as Perfect Food, Greens Plus, or Green Magma • Vegetable juice	• Diminished skin breakouts and inflammation • Plumper, smoother skin • Decreased rebound cravings and mood swings • Alleviated fibrocystic breast pain • Better sleep • Increased energy over time • Diminished under-eye puffiness • Healthier bones
Sugar Fix (Sugar includes honey, corn syrup, high-fructose corn sweeteners, grape-juice concentrate, dextrose, and other sweeteners)	• Sodas • Most bottled iced-tea drinks • Sweetened smoothies and shakes made with bananas or juice • Fruit juices • Sugar-sweetened drink mixes	• Spritzers • Unsweetened cranberry and tomato juice • Bottled drinks with low sugar content • Fruit-based (not juice-based) smoothies and shakes made with berries or papaya	• Slimmer body • More refined face shape • Clearer skin • Decreased fungal-related afflictions, such as dandruff, and sinus and yeast infections • Victory over cravings *(continued on next page)*

Your Beverage Makeovers, continued

UPGRADE YOUR	FROM	TO	BEAUTY INCENTIVES
Sugar Fix *(continued)*		• Lemonade made with healthy sweeteners • Protein shakes made with Designer Protein (natural flavor) and yogurt or kefir	• Restored alkaline balance • Prevention of wrinkles and brown (age) spots
Soda and Diet Drinks	• Sodas • Diet sodas • Powdered diet-drink mixes • Caffeinated diet drinks and sodas (see also Caffeine Fix upgrades)	• Teas and lemonade made with healthy sweetener • Spritzers • Unsweetened bottled teas (see "Better Bottled Drinks")	• Stronger bones • Fewer sugar cravings • Possible elimination of methanol-related ailments, such as headaches and vision problems (see also Sugar Fix Beauty Incentives)
Thirst Quenchers	• Sweetened iced tea • Tap water	• Teas and herbal infusions • Purified water • Spritzers	• Clearer, healthier skin • Improved body ecology and decreased consequences from sugar- or chlorine-related allergies, digestive problems, and autoimmune syndromes

UPGRADE YOUR	FROM	TO	BEAUTY INCENTIVES
Creamy Drinks	• Milk • Commercial frozen coffee drinks • Lattes • Cocoa • Sweetened smoothies and shakes made with bananas	• Soy milk • Organic 2% milk • Kefir • Lattes made with herbal coffee • Chai (unsweetened) • Cocoa Spice tea • Protein shakes made with Designer Protein (natural flavor) and yogurt or kefir	• Clearer skin • Stronger bones • Better digestion • Diminished under-eye circles and allergic responses

see the immediate and long-term benefits of upgrading your drinks. After reviewing this chart, you may want to revisit your self-inventory and write down the various upgrades you'd like to try. Then note the beauty rewards you have coming.

it's not about perfection; it's what you default to

What matters more than never doing bad things is what you default to on a regular basis. If you set up your daily routine in such a way that you have ready access to superior choices—and thus will make them on a regular basis—then the occasional times you stray from your routine aren't as important. You may have periods of backsliding on your road to palate development around the holidays or when traveling, but depending on how you prepare for those times, the degree of backsliding can be minimized.

Target Your Beauty Issues with Drinkable Herbs

	Burdock	Nettle	Green Tea	Horsetail	Ginseng	Red Clover	Chamomile	Ginger
Acne	√	√	√	√	√	√	√	√
Beauty Sleep							√	
Bones		√	√	√				
Breasts	√		√			√		
Circulation								√
Detox	√	√	√			√		√
Energy			√		√			
Hair				√				
Rashes and Inflammation	√	√	√		√	√	√	√
Nails				√				
Stress			√		√		√	
Weight			√		√			
Wrinkles			√					

Occasionally reverting to your former choices will remind you of the physical reasons you left them behind and help you appreciate how far your palate and your body have come. Eventually the benefits will replace any desire to go back.

practical strategies make all the difference

Your best intentions will inevitably be affected by convenience and practical limitations imposed by your daily routines and environment. These limitations, not willpower, are the make-or-break factors. Fortunately your intentions are easily supported with a little planning. The following tips will help you to visualize and plan a smooth transition through your first round of beverage upgrades. Once the logistics are worked out, you'll be well on your way to effortless and cumulative beauty benefits.

If you work at home all day, making changes will be relatively easy once you've gathered your initial upgrade supplies, which usually entails a trip to the health-food store. You need to prepare your upgrades in advance so they are as convenient or even more accessible than your old choices were. If you work at an office or dart around town all day, you'll need to give more thought to your strategies for heading off unhealthy, convenience-based decisions. For example, if your office kitchen has a coffeemaker full of java at an arm's reach all day, you will get nowhere with your coffee upgrades unless you plan equally convenient and tempting strategies of your own. In order to begin to create your own beauty-friendly beverage routines from this day forward, ask yourself these questions:

- Which satisfying thirst quenchers will I keep in the fridge?
- When will I make them?
- Which of my favorite brews could I carry in a thermos?
- Should I carry my own tea bags?
- Do any nearby delis carry any of the better bottled drinks (see the sidebar on page 91) or hot teas I like?

- Should I keep healthy sweetener packets with me—some in my purse, some for my desk?
- Which beverages will be on the tip of my tongue when I order at restaurants, coffeehouses, bars, or delis?
- Will I remember to order spritzers instead of soda? Tomato juice or a "Virgin Mary" instead of orange juice at brunch?
- Is there a place in town to get fresh mixed vegetable juice in the afternoon if I need an energy boost?
- Do I want to juice for myself at home? Should I buy a juicer? (See the Resources for juicers.)
- Should I buy or bring some low-carb shakes to work?

make your beverage a beautifying ritual

Consider turning your beverage habits into uplifting, self-affirming rituals. Your afternoon beverage is a good place to start. If you take some of the steps below—especially at the office—it won't be *you* who feels deprived as you indulge in your new beverage ritual.

- Choose a special place or time for your afternoon beverage ritual.
- Keep a gorgeous mug or beautiful tall glass reserved for the ritual.
- Arrange a source for pure water at work or bring bottles from home. (See the Resources for the only portable, purifying pitcher that does the job.)
- Buy a personal electric teapot for your desk or bring in a beautiful Japanese pot with matching cups. Offer tea to colleagues in intimate meetings.
- Bring in a large thermos of your favorite hot or cold brew.
- Keep your fridge (or a mini-fridge at work) filled with pure water, soy milk, organic half-and-half, cold herbal and green teas, iced Teeccino, seltzer, limes, unsweetened cranberry or pomegranate juice, and/or low-carb shakes.

- Keep your healthy sweetener packets in a beautiful, convenient container.

On your first trip to the health-food store, it may seem like you're spending more, but if you consider what you spent on your beauty-draining drinks, you may find you aren't spending more after all. Don't deprive yourself of the stuff that really makes your reflection and your life more vibrant. The dividends are high when you drink yourself beautiful.

Chapter 6

RECLAIM THE JOY OF EATING

In this chapter, you won't find any rigid rules or absolutes, and there will be no need for self-denial. (Giving up empty or fake food for real treats is not self-denial.) Rather, my approach with you—because it was the only one that worked for me—is to appeal to a long-neglected instinct deep within you: the ability to spontaneously make the wisest, most satisfying and most beautifying food choices in any given situation, based on how you feel and what your body tells you it really wants once you allow its true signals to come through. You're about to learn how to put self-denial behind you and cultivate a joyful, love–love relationship with food that will beautify your body, awaken your senses, and feed your soul with each upgrade you make. Once some informational seeds have been planted and your sensibilities have been fully recovered, your food perceptions will never be the same. But before we get to the exciting food upgrades ahead, it is important, in the spirit of shedding, to be sure there are no remaining myths or rationalizations holding you back.

Empty Foods That Make Us Look and Feel Bad

Sugar

Many nutritional experts, including the late Dr. Robert Atkins, attribute the startling rise in obesity and diabetic and pre-diabetic conditions—as much as 70 percent in the last decade in certain age groups—to the consequences of low-fat, high-sugar eating trends.

You've already heard all about sugar's cruel but seductive cycle of cravings, crashes, and weight gain, so I'll summarize the stones along the sugary trail to beauty devastation: Sugar causes insulin resistance. Sugar feeds cancer cells, which thrive on glucose. Sugar can cause varicose veins. Sugar feeds candida yeast. Sugar compromises your immune system for hours after you eat it. Sugar wrinkles your skin and ages your entire body. Sugar causes inflammation and fluid retention. Sugar raises triglyceride levels in the blood. Sugar depletes the nutrients, including chromium, that would keep you lean and stabilize your blood sugar. Sugar causes insulin to make your body store fat. I think you get it now.

White Flour

Refined flour is also a beauty and health risk. Like any refined carb, white flour is readily converted to sugar in the body. Many people who claim they don't have a sweet tooth satisfy their sugar addiction with white flour. White flour is a product of brilliant PR and the profit motives of food manufacturers. Everything of value is taken from a wheat kernel, such as the wheat germ, minerals, antioxidants, vital oils, and crucial fiber. Then the flour is bleached, and sometimes even preserved, leaving traces of carcinogens like formaldehyde. The resulting substance is then promoted like it was the best thing since . . .

white bread! Eating refined flour and anything made with it on a regular basis cumulatively damages, depletes, and deprives your precious body.

Hydrogenated Fat

It surprises me that people still use margarine or still don't know about hydrogenated fat—one of the most dangerous foods we can eat and an ingredient the FDA has assured us is food even though it does not fit even the broadest definition. Its harmfulness is now undisputed.

Hydrogenated fat is used to "embalm" packaged foods to extend their shelf life. Also known as trans-fatty acids, or trans-fats, this substance assaults your body with free radicals every time you eat it. Free radicals are potentially toxic molecules that are thought to play an important role in the development of many serious diseases, including heart disease, cancer, and Alzheimer's disease. According to Udo Erasmus, Ph.D., author of *Fats That Heal, Fats That Kill*, trans-fats take the place of precious essential fatty acids (EFAs) and other real fats in the cells and wreak havoc on all kinds of processes, influencing hormone activity and causing inflammation.

In 2003 the FDA made a requirement that food manufacturers list the amount of trans-fats on food labels. This still gives the impression that this substance is food, but the truth is that there is no acceptable or safe level of daily intake of trans-fats.

Additives, Preservatives, and "Excitotoxins"

Additives can be in foods in such seemingly insignificant amounts that it's hard to imagine they could do us much harm. Used by manufacturers to extend shelf life and manipulate texture or flavor for minimal cost, they seem harmless enough, but some may trigger allergic reactions, headaches, and even long-term neurological problems.

Sulfites, commonly found in wines, dried fruit, and salad-bar foods, are sometimes used to preserve food at restaurants, where the law requires a posted notice of its use, although this law is often unheeded. Sulfites trigger mild to severe reactions in sensitive people, as can monosodium glutamate (MSG), known as an excitotoxin because it can overstimulate brain cells and trigger migraines, according to Russell L. Blaylock, M.D., author of *Excitotoxins: The Taste That Kills.* "Hydrolyzed vegetable protein" is just another alias for MSG and is found in canned and prepared foods and gravy mixes. Nitrates in bacon and other cured meats are carcinogens. Red dye #3, used in maraschino cherries, fruit cocktail, and some baked goods, has been shown to cause thyroid tumors in rats, according to a 1983 review committee report requested by the FDA.

If it never goes bad, it can't make you beautiful.

What we don't know about food additives may be even scarier than what we do know. It's best to avoid them. The healthiest, most revitalizing foods spoil the quickest. If it never goes bad, it was never good to begin with. And it can't make you beautiful.

Fat-Free Foods

Years ago, after overcoming my eating disorder, I watched Dr. John MacDougall and Dr. Barry Sears duke it out about their respective popular diets. Hearing MacDougall's low-fat recommendations was like a flashback to my compulsive past. For more than a decade, my cupboards were stocked with "damage-control" diet foods like fat-free soups and shake mixes, air-popped popcorn, and rice cakes. Throughout the 1990s, after my recovery, I started to see this all-you-can-eat-of-nothing approach—which I came up with out of desperation from my disease—being recommended by registered dieticians everywhere as an ongoing way to eat, as if it were *healthy.* On the contrary, low-fat eating can, in some cases, even cause the chemical relationship with food that leads to food obsession, even in the absence of a severe emotional problem.

In summer of 2002, the *New York Times* published Gary Taubes's powerful expose of the workings behind the low-fat myth, "What If It's All Been a Big Fat Lie?" which caused a stir throughout the mainstream nutritional community by spotlighting the complete lack of evidence in support of low-fat eating as well as the basic science that points to its dangers. Taubes

---

MYTH: *A calorie is a calorie.*

TRUTH: *It's not the calorie count; it's the calorie kind.*

Insisting that a calorie is like any other calorie is like saying two songs sound the same because they're both three minutes long. Controlling calorie intake without considering the caloric *form* can leave you deeply deprived of true sustenance while turning your body into a fat-storing machine. One food can set you up for cravings, weight gain, and energy slumps, while the caloric equivalent of another food can leave you energized and slim. In his book *The Zone*, Dr. Barry Sears explains how even fat-free foods can cause insulin to increase fat storage in the body, and he refers to a landmark study published in the *Lancet* nearly fifty years ago which showed that patients eating high-fat diets lost significant weight while the high-carb eaters on *the same number of calories* lost none. The glycemic index, nutrient density, fiber content, and hormone response as well as order and combination of what you eat and even the supplements you consume with foods have much more impact on your ultimate shape and radiance than calories or fat grams.

interviewed both mainstream and "renegade" diet experts and made crystal clear what some of us have known or suspected for years: Not only is low-fat not the answer, it may well be the *problem*. America's fat consumption went down for the first time in the '80s and '90s, and correspondingly, obesity statistics skyrocketed. And all the while, the United States Department of Agriculture, the American Dietetic Association, the

MYTH: *A nutritionist is a nutritionist is a nutritionist.*

TRUTH: *Nutritionists who are focused on calories and fat grams won't address your deeper issues.*

Clinical—as opposed to holistic—nutrition still largely discounts the role of food and supplements as healing tools, and it has only begun to acknowledge them as the proven disease-preventing tools they are. It continues to downplay the distinction between fresh, whole foods and dead foods containing antinutrients like hydrogenated fats.

Is your nutritionist hip? If you're getting talk about calories, egg-white omelets, dry bagels, fat grams, RDAs, or the Food Guide Pyramid and not much else, you're not getting healing, beautifying information.

American Heart Association, and the American Medical Association, along with most nutritionists in this country, perpetuated the low-fat myth, despite having no evidence to support it and proof that it may actually contribute to heart disease and obesity.

the solution: become a food snob

Food is not beauty's enemy. Fake food is. It assaults your body and desensitizes your tastes while sensitizing your skin, sapping your vitality, and creating imbalances and cravings that can't be satisfied. Say no to beauty poison. Start turning your nose up at fake food. Eat only live, fresh, perishable foods. Beware of denatured, hydrogenated, overcooked, and indefinitely preserved foods.

stop eating light and start eating *well*

It's not about eating light; it's about eating well. Quality is far more important than quantity. No one likes to feel deprived. But eating empty "virtual food"—now *that's* deprivation. Or even worse: It can be cellular starvation and poisoning combined. The USDA's low-fat, high-carb recommendations and its lack of emphasis on the quality of food make it easy to rationalize unhealthy eating habits and bury yourself under the Food Guide Pyramid. Over the last twenty years the number of overweight Americans has nearly doubled as more Americans have been seduced into using food as a drug and once addicted, many people cling to fat-free and no-calorie tactics to keep from becoming obese since they can't stop eating empty foods.

Those of us who grew up on packaged foods, iceberg-lettuce salads, and white rice eat them because they're easily available and familiar. The term "health food" conjures images of scary, weird-tasting grub with crude textures and colors. Americans like their uniformly textured bread and pure whites—rice, potatoes, and pasta. Beyond sweetness or saltiness, they don't want any taste surprises. The French secret to staying slim and avoiding heart disease while eating rich foods is not the wine. The French do not live on packaged, hydrogenated food. They eat all kinds of cheese and fat, and they eat fresh produce that may not look as pretty as ours, but it tastes much better and contains more nutrients. Fashion models I've worked with who work in Europe and then return to the United States always complain that they can eat more and yet lose weight while abroad but that they gain weight and don't feel as well while eating less once they've returned here.

> *MYTH:* **A beautiful body means deprivation and the end of decadence.**
>
> *TRUTH:* **A beautiful body means the end of deprivation and the beginning of a new kind of decadence: pure, real food.**

Many people think of decadence as "letting go" and bingeing on fake foods that start their body and mind on a roller coaster of chemical cravings and emotional guilt. They consider a full plate of full-fat, nutrient-dense, freshly prepared food off limits or extravagant. But every person—and every *body*—deserves such treatment. And you won't believe what it can do for your looks, your spirit, and your relationship with food.

Here's a taste of decadence: Plump blackberries in organic, full-fat yogurt; sugar-free Belgian dark chocolate; delicate organic baby lettuces or locally grown, hand-picked heirloom tomatoes drizzled with walnut oil; exotic mushrooms and fresh herbs; arugula and goat cheese with slices of exotic pears; crisp wedges of Granny Smith apples dipped in raw, organic almond butter; organic black mission figs covered with thick Greek yogurt; free-range chicken sausage with sage and apples; ripe avocado slices, laced with Scotch Bonnet Hot Sauce, on moist, sprouted, nutty, seedy, meal-worthy bread. I hope I'm making your mouth water. I defy you to wolf down foods such as these. They *make* you slow down. I've been known to moan with delight while eating these foods. Treat yourself to the most decadent foods in the world. Giving up the old empty foods will easily offset the cost.

get gorgeous by going low-glycemic

The technical term for the kind of eating that makes us beautiful is eating "low-glycemic." The glycemic index (GI) is a measure of a food's impact on blood-sugar levels in the body. In general, high-glycemic foods are based on white flour or sugar, such as pasta, starchy vegetables (for example, potatoes and corn), and conventional candies, desserts, and baked goods. Even some whole grains, if eaten by themselves or in large quantities, can set off the cycle of elevated insulin, cravings, and weight gain similar to the consequences of insulin resistance discussed in the previous chapter. You can only escape this "carbohydrate hell"—as Dr. Sears calls it—by making the switch to low-glycemic eating. Low-glycemic foods cause a slower rise in blood-sugar levels than high-glycemic foods and tend to be low in sugar but higher in protein, fat, fiber, and beneficial nutrients that satisfy the body longer and more authentically. As a result, the body begins to express true hunger again rather than being led by the swinging pendulum of blood-sugar-induced cravings.

The lower a meal's GI rating, the kinder it is to your body and skin, the more slimming it is, and the more stable your moods, energy, and blood-sugar levels. By avoiding high-glycemic foods—which requires zero deprivation once you learn about their low-carb equivalents—you can decrease your risk of heart disease and possibly even reverse some symptoms of diabetes.

If you are interested in learning more about the glycemic index, there are numerous books you can consult (see the Resources). The University of Sydney's GI Web site, *www.glycemicindex.com*, is a great place to start. You may find it interesting to check out the numbers to get a sense of how a potato compares with whole-wheat pasta, for example, but I really don't suggest counting the GIs of everything you eat.

Frankly, I have never counted GIs myself. I fell upon low-glycemic eating—a term I find a bit tiring, since this is basically just real-food eating—

quite by accident, not by following a diet. About ten years ago I was stuck in a hotel room after room service had ended, and I pondered the choices in the mini-bar. "Candy or nuts?" I debated in anguish, having long since relegated both to my "bad food" list. I chose the nuts. The next morning, I was flabbergasted to feel fantastic and flatter in the stomach. From there my experiments with fat increased, and I started to butter my whole-grain toast and eat eggs and yogurt instead of cereal for breakfast. I said good-bye to the former energy lulls from eating whole grains without fat. There's something powerful about learning to sense which foods are best and honing your natural instincts.

If you never want to look at a GI chart, you will do just fine with the upgrades I suggest in the pages ahead, which have lower GI factored in for you along with other important issues like nutrient density and, particularly, taste. I am confident that your body will get used to and learn to detect foods which do and don't throw its chemistry off-balance and that you'll come to prefer these upgraded foods.

Clever Combining Heightens the Appeal of a Meal While Minimizing Its Glycemic Impact

It's always a good idea to start a meal with protein or fat, such as a nibble of cheese—as opposed to wine or bread on an empty stomach—so you don't immediately shock your system into pumping out too much insulin. But a food's GI isn't the last word on whether or not you should allow that food into your life. It actually might restrict you unnecessarily if you don't account for the fact that you can combine and average foods of various GIs to create a low-impact meal.

For people who don't have carb cravings, foods containing whole-grain flour might be eaten without trouble if combined with low-GI foods like protein, fiber, or fat, all of which lower the overall glycemic index of any meal. If you just gradually upgrade your meal components to lower-glycemic choices and combinations, the relationship with food that nature had always intended for you to have will finally unfold.

The incredible thing is that low-glycemic combinations make meals and snacks more satisfying. Consider low-carb tortilla chips and organic cheese for your nachos, organic and free-range meats and dairy to garnish and add flavor to your meals, and non-hydrogenated nut butters for your celery. Pure decadence!

With today's new protein-based pastas, cereals, and low-carb chips and chocolate, you can eat all of the old favorites and use these increasingly

> **MYTH: *Eating high-cholesterol foods causes heart disease.***
>
> **TRUTH: *High-glycemic foods can cause heart problems.***
>
> Repeated large-scale studies (including a 2002 study of 12,553 men published in the *American Journal of Cardiology*) have failed to confirm that dietary cholesterol (such as eating eggs) has any significant impact on serum-cholesterol levels, let alone heart disease. On the other hand, it is now known that high-glycemic foods and related problems like insulin resistance *can* cause obesity and raise triglycerides, posing much more danger to your heart.

available foods as invaluable tools to get and keep you free of the effects of high-glycemic foods. You will begin to recognize foods that drag you down or drug you, and you can make a mental note to eliminate, upgrade, or combine those foods with more fat, fiber, or protein. In this way, your body will begin to do the counting for you.

is organic food worth the price?

You'll rarely see quantity discounts on real, and particularly organic, foods because they have genuine value. But the recent increase in sales of organic foods and products is a sign that consumers are making—and paying for—the honest distinction between organic and conventionally produced products; however, some people aren't clear about why organic products are good for you. One woman said to me, "I bought some organic yogurt, and I was surprised that it was so sweet!" Organic doesn't necessarily mean healthy. There are all sorts of sugar-laden, white flour–based organic products that could still be detrimental to your health. But eating organic will always spare you needless chemicals while doing something important for the health of our planet and, very likely, the future security of our food supply. They don't call organic "sustainable agriculture" for nothing.

So what exactly is organic? In 2002 the USDA finally standardized the requirements for use of the term *organic*. Under the regulation, all products labeled as organic must be produced without hormones, antibiotics, pesticides, synthetic fertilizers including sewage sludge, irradiation, or genetically modified ingredients. Organic meat must come from animals which eat only organic feed that hasn't been treated with hormones or antibiotics. The animals must also have access to the outdoors with protection from excessive heat and cold when needed. In other words, they must be treated humanely. Learning about organic foods opens your eyes to the unappealing methods used to produce conventional foods.

Biodynamic farming is a higher form of organic agriculture that takes even greater care in harvesting and preserving precious nutrients.

Six Reasons to Buy Organic

No Pesticides

If you eat meat and dairy products and can buy only a few organic items, make meat and dairy products the ones you buy organic. According to the

EPA, the majority of all pesticide residues are found in meat, poultry, and dairy products. Residues from chemicals and pesticides in grass or grain feed are largely stored in an animal's fat. Likewise, certain pesticides we take in from these conventionally produced animal products, fruits, and vegetables can accumulate in the human body, mimicking hormones and challenging the immune system. Some toxicologists believe we may even accumulate fat to keep such toxins away from our vital organs.

No Growth Hormones

The problems with meat and dairy are man-made, not the fault of nature. Recombinant Bovine Growth Hormone (rBGH), a genetically modified drug, has been injected into conventional dairy cows since it was approved in 1993 despite warnings against such approval by the General Accounting Office; the Consumer Policy Institute of the Consumers Union, the nonprofit group that publishes *Consumer Reports* magazine; and countless other consumer and environmental groups.

IGF-1, a key growth hormone that has been linked to breast and prostate cancers, may have a greater presence in hormone-treated meats and dairy. In addition to the unknown risks to humans, there are known consequences of rBGH on both the cows and the foods we eat. Because one of the common side effects of rBGH is mastitis (udder infection), additional antibiotics must be used in conventional milk production. The antibiotics and pus from the infection are commonly introduced into milk as a result of the infections. I'll bet that extra dollar you didn't want to pay for organic milk doesn't sound so unreasonable now.

No Antibiotics

In the early 1990s, *Consumer Reports* tested milk samples and found fifty-two different antibiotics commonly used to treat mastitis in cows. The Union of Concerned Scientists, a nonprofit group in Washington, D.C., estimated that more antibiotics are used to treat healthy animals in the United States than sick humans. Antibiotics are also widely used as growth promoters in conventional meat production and—many farmers believe—as a substitute for sanitary conditions and thorough inspections. This practice is of great concern among scientists and government agencies because such overuse of antibiotics can give rise to strains of drug-resistant bacteria.

For more information and documentation on antibiotics and rBGH in dairy, poultry, and meat production, contact the Consumer Policy Institute of the Consumers Union (see the Resources).

No Irradiation

Foods are irradiated to kill microorganisms and stop the ripening process. Irradiation has been shown to

- Reduce nutrients in food
- Halt enzyme activity in food, which the body needs
- Form toxic by-products, such as benzene and formaldehyde
- Cause chemicals used on the food to form completely new, foreign chemicals called unique radiolytic products (URPs) with unknown effects

No Sewage Sludge

Instead of the compost used in organic farming, conventional foods in the United States can be grown in a mudlike by-product from sewage-treatment plants, which, because it was considered hazardous, was banned by the government in the early 1990s from being dumped into oceans. Aside from the sheer disgustingness of the concept, the problem is that industrial and domestic hazardous waste and chemicals survive the sewage-treatment process. In 1990, the EPA stated that sewage sludge "may include volatiles, organic solids, nutrients, disease-causing pathogenic organisms, heavy metals, inorganic ions, and toxic organic chemicals from industrial wastes, household chemicals, and pesticides."

No Genetically Modified Organisms

Unlike the citizens of most other countries, Americans are largely unaware that much of the food they eat contains GMOs. Nor are they aware of what impact these modifications may have on their health or that of the planet, largely because this information is not widely publicized. Field and lab tests reported by the Organic Consumers Association show that

- GMOs have caused farmers to use two to five times more herbicides than in conventional seed farming.
- GMOs have created antibiotic-resistant genes. These genes are found in all GMOs. A study by researchers at the University of Newcastle-upon-Tyne showed that GMOs can transfer DNA into the bacteria of the digestive tract so that animals and humans ingesting GMOs are likely to incubate increasingly virulent pathogens as well as antibiotic-resistant organisms. (Until this recent study, the makers of GMOs denied this possibility.)
- GMOs have been found to yield herbicide-resistant super-weeds in Canada.
- GMOs have shifted delicate ecological balances so that formerly minor pests are becoming major problems. In 1999, researchers at Cornell University found that pollen from genetically modified corn was poisonous to monarch butterflies, while in a British study, rats fed genetically modified potatoes suffered damage to their vital organs and immune systems.

ORGANIC, DELIVERED ANYWHERE

If you live in a town that doesn't offer many organic products, don't despair. A handful of companies deliver fresh organic produce just about anywhere in the country (see the Resources).

why grass-fed is best

Not all organic animals are grass-fed, but grass-fed organic cows and chicks make healthier meat and dairy products. They have been found to contain healthy nutrients that have all but disappeared from conventional meats, such as omega-3 fatty acids and conjugated linolenic acid (CLA), which has been shown to promote fat loss and possibly prevent cancer. Grass-fed cows have up to five times more CLA than cows raised on the standard industry diet. Most recently it was found that CLA supplements may even diminish cellulite and decrease thigh circumference when used in conjunction with certain herbal combinations.

when your body treats a food as a toxin

There is one last consideration to take into account before embarking on your food upgrades: You may know about your food allergies, but what about your food sensitivities? In his book *Your Hidden Food Allergies Are Making You Fat* (Prima Publishing, 1998), Rudy Rivera, M.D., explains that when left undiagnosed, hidden allergies produce a much wider range of subtle symptoms, including weight gain. According to Dr. Susan Lark, edema (fluid retention) and even fat accumulation can result from eating foods you are sensitive to. She recommends that women note typical signs of sensitivity, which include headache, increased heart rate, diarrhea, bloating, and low energy. She also recommends eliminating typical sensitizing foods such as wheat, dairy, corn, soy, and eggs and then adding them back one by one over a couple of weeks to determine your sensitivities. See the Resources for information on the ALCAT test, one of the most sensitive blood tests for determining food sensitivities.

your kitchen-cabinet makeover

A makeover of the contents of your kitchen cabinet (and refrigerator) is like a sculptor acquiring a new set of raw materials. Your final creation of yourself can be an entirely different work of art. The Kitchen-Cabinet Makeover is a series of pro–beauty food upgrades that, once in place, will effortlessly begin to transform your body and your skin while delighting your tastes. The idea is to find practical, accessible upgrades that suit both your palate and your lifestyle. The suggested upgrades in the pages ahead are mostly available through health-food stores. Ordering information for hard-to-find products is listed in the Resources. If you have a health condition, get approval from your doctor before changing your diet.

For the first few weeks the goal will be to identify and upgrade your favorite staples—your autopilot choices. As you upgrade your foods, moving from depleted and denatured foods to body-decadent pleasures, the biggest shift will be moving food out of your cabinets and putting more into your refrigerator. For example, the best beauty-enhancing breads are the ones that should be refrigerated and are only good for a day or two. And, of course, fresh produce can revitalize your body, while canned will not.

resensitize your taste buds gradually

The best upgrades are the ones that don't feel like substitutions after only a few days. Don't deny your tastes. Here's something else to consider: Before you pass final judgment on the taste of any food, your taste buds may need to recover from years of overstimulation from oversalted and oversweetened foods, so don't get ahead of the process. Once resensitized, your taste buds will regain the ability to recognize and appreciate the wide varieties of subtle flavors available in real foods. Finally, don't accept second-rate substitutions. There's a healthy way to satisfy each and every craving. Your changing sensibilities will soon compel you to choose foods you may never have dreamed you'd prefer.

clear out the cupboards for your kitchen-cabinet makeover

For those of you who are partially or fully addicted to sugar and carbs, I strongly and compassionately advise you to throw out all forms of these drugs by emptying your kitchen cabinets of the sugar, flour, white pasta, and refined anything. If you binge on whole-grain breads or pasta, ditch those, too, and start clean with all low-carb upgrades. You will go through a brief withdrawal period, but the carb claws won't lose their grip unless you part with grains at least temporarily. If you are not a carb addict, you can hang on to the brown rice and other whole grains and breads that

LINDA: CRAVINGS LIFTED IN ONE DAY

This letter is from a woman who came to one of my programs:

Dear Kat: I attended your workshop this past weekend and I again want to say thank you!

Preceding the workshop, my sugar addiction (my "demon") was out of control. I was bingeing continuously but couldn't do anything about it.

I went to the grocery store on my way home from your workshop and had no interest in any baked goods, candy, or sweets. I realized that I had no cravings at all. The only way I can explain it is that the quality of the foods we were served during the day chemically removed my cravings. My body was so ready for this! I haven't had a craving since, and I am enjoying delicious meals and snacks following your principles and have tremendous energy. It seems like a miracle to me. I also plan to continue my transformation beyond my diet. I am taking supplements and will change out my skin-care, hair-care, and makeup products at my first opportunity. Thank you for showing me the way to my own transformation. You are a miracle worker!

—Linda Q.
Atlanta, Georgia

meet the criteria below and eat them in lower glycemic combinations. With the other delicious upgrades, your transition will be nearly painless, and you will feel and see changes in the mirror in only a few days. The next step is to stock up on—and stick with—your low-impact upgrades. As you read on, jot down the upgrades you'd like to try in your self-inventory notebook.

upgrading your breads, bagels, and buns

If you feel you have a sane relationship with bread and plan on keeping it around, find good, whole-grain, preferably higher-protein breads—not the feeble, caramel-colored, hydrogenated offerings dubiously dubbed

A BETTER CEREAL

Uncle Sam cereal has remained unchanged since 1908. It's simple (even in its packaging) and unsweetened, and the taste of the wheat is uncommonly vibrant to the evolved palate. It is low-glycemic and packed with flax-seeds that deliver a whopping 2,000 mg of skin-beautifying and body-loving essential omega-3 fatty acids per serving (be sure to chew well to liberate the oils in the seeds). It costs much less than the brightly packaged "candy" that comes in most other cereal boxes. Try it with unsweetened soy milk and a scoop of whey protein powder or on top of plain yogurt with berries. Palates-in-training can use a little healthy sweetener.

"wheat bread." (Note that wheat flour is the same as white flour.) Only 100 percent whole grain is the real thing. Look for dark, dense, moist, and grainy real bread that needs refrigeration and only lasts a couple of days. (You can freeze half of it to make it last.) Real whole-grain, nutty, seeded breads taste moist and delicious on their own, but again, they are better for you if eaten with fat or protein, such as almond butter, avocado slices, or olive oil. The glycemic level is further lowered and the combination is more of a meal. Look in your health-food store's refrigerated section for low-carb breads, flourless breads, or breads with sprouted grains. See the Resources for some standouts, and keep testing them until you find some you like.

EFFECTIVE CARB LISTINGS

"Effective carbs" is a term you'll see on low-carb food labels. Due to their molecular structure, certain fibers and sweeteners are considered low-impact carbs because they are not absorbed. Manufacturers determine the number of effective carbs by subtracting carbs that have little or no blood-sugar impact from the total carb count of a food.

LOW-CARB CONNOISSEUR'S PASTA CHOICE

Keto Spaghetti is the first convincing low-carb pasta I have tasted. It has only 5 grams of effective carbs, compared with the blood-sugar-spiking 35 to 40 grams you get with white and even whole-grain pastas. Remember to always cook pasta al dente (firm), which keeps the glycemic index lower, and add oil or a protein. Pesto works well.

UPGRADE YOUR SWEET FIX

Denatured or Depleted Choice	Pro-Beauty Choice	Body-Decadent Splurge
• Standard chocolate, ice cream, cookies, cakes, donuts, pastries, and candy	• Low-carb chocolate • Low-carb cookies • Low-carb cake • Low-fat or regular (but not nonfat!) yogurt with berries and a sprinkling of unsweetened Uncle Sam cereal, soy-nut granola, Soy Nutlettes, or other low-glycemic crunch • Low-carb cheesecake	• Organic Belgian dark, maltitol, or Splenda-sweetened chocolate • Homemade ice cream made with healthy sweetener and real vanilla bean, chocolate, or coconut milk (see sidebar below) • Homemade hot chocolate made with organic whole milk or soy milk, real cocoa, and healthy sweetener

HOMEMADE LOW-CARB ICE CREAM AND SORBETS

The Vitamix 5000, a one-of-a-kind industrial kitchen appliance, turns rock-hard frozen peaches or berries into super-smooth sorbet in seconds. It makes incredible smoothies, grinds flaxseeds, and even grinds flour right from grains, dried legumes, or seeds. I have made incredible organic chocolate, green tea, and "mocha" ice cream from Teeccino, frozen coconut milk cubes, organic frozen milk cubes, and a touch of healthy sweetener. In addition, I have ground buckwheat, added buttermilk, and poured pancakes right from the machine. It is expensive, but you will use it so often that it will pay itself off in no time (see the Resources).

UPGRADE YOUR FRUITS

Get creative with fruit: use tart berries, exotic pears, apples, or orange slices in your salads, smoothies, and sorbets. Try heated, mashed berries over low-carb pancakes.

Denatured or Depleted Choice	Pro-Beauty Choice	Body-Decadent Splurge
• Canned fruit • Fruit juices (see beverage upgrades for taste-evolving alternatives) • Dried fruit	• Fresh, whole, nutrient-dense and deep- or brightly colored fruits, such as blackberries, blueberries, raspberries, cranberries, strawberries, cantaloupe, watermelon, papaya, plums, peaches, and mangoes	• Organic fresh or frozen berries • Fresh Black Mission figs dipped in organic, full-fat, or Greek yogurt • Red currants, champagne grapes, exotic pears, pomegranates, or papaya with fresh mint

BEAUTIFYING BERRIES

Fresh berries in season are not only a luscious splurge but perhaps the most impressive fruits of all when you consider their glycemic index, high nutrient density, high fiber content, taste, and versatility. Try throwing blueberries into yogurt or even over a salad. Berries contain phytochemicals that beautify the skin and also inhibit cervical and breast cancer in cultured cells, according to a May 2001 study reported by the USDA Research Service.

UPGRADE YOUR VEGETABLES

Use lots of herbs, like garlic, ginger, or lemon wedges, as well as toasted nuts and high-quality finishing oils, such as roasted sesame, walnut, or chili oils, for ethnic variation and to make your vegetable dishes savory and aromatic.

Denatured or Depleted Choice	Pro-Beauty Choice	Body-Decadent Splurge
• Iceberg lettuce • Canned vegetables • Potatoes and corn	• Fresh spinach or romaine lettuce—the darker the better • Fresh peppers, parsley (tabouli is the best way to get more of this), broccoli, sugar snaps, snow peas, asparagus, tomatoes, and avocados • Frozen green vegetables (if the fresh vegetable is not in season)	• Organic mesclun greens • Baby spinach • Arugula • Watercress • Shiitake and other exotic mushrooms • Yellow and red peppers • Fresh herbs • Frozen organic vegetables (if the fresh vegetable is not in season)

Beauty tip: If you really want to glow, eat some raw vegetables every day for the enzymes, which fight inflammation, allergies, and skin flare-ups. Cooking and pasteurization kills vital enzymes in food.

DESIGN A DECADENT MEAL SALAD

Forget iceberg lettuce, hydrogenated croutons, and bottled dressing. This truly decadent salad is a higher sensory experience and a whole meal in itself:

- Dark, organic greens such as arugula, watercress, baby spinach, or mesclun greens
- Red onion
- Apple or pear slices
- Fresh blue cheese, feta, or Gorgonzola or alternative protein choices such as avocado, goat cheese, hard-boiled eggs, chicken, or tuna
- Toasted or plain walnuts or other nuts or seeds, such as pumpkin
- Cold-pressed gourmet oil, such as extra virgin olive, grapeseed, walnut, or pumpkinseed oils, and balsamic vinegar

Greens and Your Bones

Greens may be even more effective than dairy at building bones. Vitamin K, found in large amounts in greens, was once primarily thought of as a blood-clotting agent, but now it has been discovered to be a major contributor to bone health. Oils and fats on your salad enhance the absorption of vitamin K.

UPGRADE YOUR OILS, DRESSINGS, AND CONDIMENTS

Infuse foods with herbs and the finest oils for rejuvenation and sensual indulgence. Your basic major-brand corn, canola, sunflower, and safflower oils are generally bleached and oxidized and may contain hexane residues. For cooking, you want oils that don't break down with heat. For high-temperature cooking, such as stir-frying, the healthiest oil may be grapeseed, which doesn't peroxidize at higher temperatures and raises the "good" and lowers the "bad" cholesterol.

Denatured or Depleted Choice	Pro-Beauty Choice	Body-Decadent Splurge
• Common bleached cooking oils • Hydrogenated shortenings • Margarine • Bottled salad dressings, spreads, and dips • Soy sauce	• Cold-pressed grapeseed oil • Extra virgin olive oil • Roasted sesame and chili oils • Organic butter (or ghee for the lactose-intolerant) • Bragg's Liquid Aminos instead of soy sauce *For high-temperature cooking:* • Grapeseed oil • Unrefined coconut oil	• Exotic cold-pressed finishing oils: sesame, walnut, Austrian pumpkin seed, and truffle-infused olive oil • Organic flaxseed oil (therapeutic to your hair, skin, and heart, but very perishable, so don't cook with it and keep it in the fridge or freezer to preserve its benefits)

UPGRADE YOUR DAIRY

Dairy tips: Unlike U.S. cheeses, most European cheeses do not contain growth hormones and antibiotic residues. Be aware that experts on Mad Cow Disease continue to advise the avoidance of meat and dairy products wherever rendered animal parts have been used in livestock feed (including the United States and Great Britain).

Denatured or Depleted Choice	Pro-Beauty Choice	Body-Decadent Splurge
• Conventionally produced milk and milk products • Nonfat milk • Sweetened yogurt • Processed cheese	• Organic low-fat and regular plain yogurt • Kefir • Goat milk • Soy milk and soy yogurt • Natural cheese	• Organic butter • Biodynamic yogurt • Organic cheese

SAFER GRILLING WITH STRATEGIC MARINADES

Grilling meats can form carcinogens called heterocyclic amines (HCAs); however, some eye-opening studies comparing sweet Western barbeque sauces with Asian antioxidant-containing marinades showed that the Western honey-based marinades increased dangerous HCAs (sugar does it again!), while Asian and tumeric- and garlic-based marinades *reduced* HCAs. Also note that consumption of green tea helps block HCAs. So don't give up the barbeque; just do it smarter!

UPGRADE YOUR PROTEIN

Eating protein with every meal and snack is the best way to keep yourself off the pendulum. And now that formerly high-carb foods are being made with more protein, the low-glycemic choices are becoming endless and can fulfill any comfort food yearning without high-carb consequences.

Denatured or Depleted Choice	Pro-Beauty Choice	Body-Decadent Splurge
• Conventionally raised or cured meats and poultry • Frozen breaded or fried fish • Canned or processed roasted nuts and seeds • Hydrogenated, processed peanut butter • Canned refried or baked beans	• Free-range meat and poultry • Fresh, omega-3 fat-rich fish, such as salmon • Avocado • Fresh unroasted nuts: walnuts, almonds, Brazil nuts, and soy nuts • Pumpkin- and flaxseeds • Natural almond and soy nut butters • Sesame tahini • Canned soybeans • Chicken sausage and ground turkey	• Wild Alaskan salmon • Free-range, nitrate-free bacon (or turkey bacon) • Protein based low-carb pastas, cereals, and munchies

nuts and seeds: the ultimate beauty food

Nuts and seeds are "it" for health, taste, and beauty benefits for the skin and body. A handful of Brazil nuts pack a day's worth of selenium. Almonds and sesame seeds are high in calcium. Almonds and walnuts both lower LDL cholesterol. Walnuts raise serotonin levels. The omega-3s in flax and walnuts add luster to the skin and hair. Hummus and sesame tahini are full of calcium. Instead of bread with your hummus, try Cracker Flax, a cracker made out of flaxseeds that tastes surprisingly good (see the Resources).

NUT TRICKS

Buy a nut mixture at the health-food store and toss it with a few roasted, tamarind-seasoned almonds or spicy seasoned pumpkinseeds; they make the whole mix even tastier. Put nuts on salads, in yogurt, and in whole-grain pilafs.

An article in the American Heart Association's publication *Circulation* suggested that people trying to maintain heart health should eat almonds as part of a balanced diet. A University of Toronto clinical trial found that eating one ounce of almonds a day lowered LDL cholesterol. Be sure to store nuts in tightly sealed containers and refrigerate them so they don't oxidize, which produces by-products (lipid peroxides) that may accelerate the aging process.

---

fabulous fatty fish

Deep-sea, cold-water fish is one of the best sources of omega-3 EFAs, which are great for your heart, your skin, and everything in between. Salmon is one of the foods highest in omega-3 fatty acids. In *The Perricone Prescription*, Dr. Perricone asserts that the DMAE in salmon firms the skin by raising levels of key neurochemicals.

Cold-water fish such as salmon, mackerel, herring, and sardines are great beauty food, but avoid farm-raised fish, which is not a good source of EFAs and is rarely pure. Farm-raised fish is often artificially colored with feed additives, treated with antibiotics because of unsanitary conditions, and higher in pesticides. Environmental groups advocate wild Alaskan salmon (not Atlantic salmon, which is usually farmed) as the most sustainable variety. Fish sustainability is very fragile and ever-changing, so it is important to ask questions at the fish market and be wary of culinary trends that could wipe out certain species. You can have wild Alaskan salmon and other premium sustainable fish delivered to you anywhere in the country (see the Resources).

SPICE IT UP: INDULGE YOUR SENSES AND YOUR BODY

Nothing elevates a dish to gourmet, mouth-watering status more easily and healthily than herbs and spices. Two of my favorite tricks are adding fennel seed to ground turkey to give it that savory Italian sausage taste and adding a pinch of tarragon to my scrambled eggs for a touch of buttery sweetness. Just about every spice studied has been found to have unique health properties, including antibacterial and antifungal actions. In hot climates where refrigeration is scarce, people of many cultures, such as those in India, have depended on spices like curry to preserve food. (Please don't try that at home!) Spices such as cayenne have also been shown in recent research to reduce the appetite and increase satiety and well-being after a meal.

- **Garlic** is a potent antibiotic that has been reported to lower cholesterol in some cases.
- **Cayenne**, especially in a topical form, has been shown to relieve pain. There is strong evidence that it can relieve cluster headaches, heartburn, and indigestion (though people with this condition should use it cautiously) and help obesity.
- **Ginger** improves digestion, eases nausea, improves circulation, and is being researched as a heart tonic.

- **Turmeric**, a component of Indian curry, has shown potent anti-inflammatory, anticancer, and liver-protective benefits in numerous studies. It was also recently shown to block the absorption of estrogen-mimicking chemicals, nitrosamines from processed meats, and even radiation to varying degrees.
- **Cilantro**, in a study using cilantro pesto, has been shown to detoxify heavy metals by carrying them out of the body.
- **Cinnamon** has shown antibacterial activity, and one of its active components demonstrated improved sugar metabolism in a USDA study.

These tidbits are just the tip of the iceberg. Stunning benefits are just now being identified and studied for nearly every fresh herb, cold-pressed oil, and spice you can think of. So the next time you find yourself saying, "Everything that tastes good is bad for you," stop yourself. Life is good when you spice it up!

get into cooking if you can

Consider cooking at home more often and celebrating at home with simple, real food. Express your creativity and your passion for creating yourself and your impact on the lives of everyone you cook for with the food you prepare. Plan your menu based on what looks really good at the market rather than sticking with a rigid list. Choose your raw materials with passionate discernment. Treat the food delicately. Boiling vegetables will deplete most nutrients, while steaming or roasting will preserve more of them. Peeling also robs vegetables of some of their most potent benefits, so try scrubbing instead. Be a connoisseur—not only of the food you're creating but of the beauty you are creating with that food.

be high-maintenance: stand up for your body and your beauty

If demanding real food is being high-maintenance, then by all means, be high-maintenance. Remember, convenience and strategy really count. You'll need to rally your resources and go through a little logistical adjustment period before your new choices become automatic. This is particularly true if food availability in your area is limited. Real food should be just as accessible as a restroom, running water, or any form of basic self-care, and you should assert your need for it without apology. By doing so, you will join a new wave of consumer awareness and demand that is bringing better food to markets and restaurants everywhere.

Once you become accustomed to true sustenance, your body will demand it as it fulfills a deep need like no brightly packaged, hydrogenated piece of technology ever could.

Chapter 7

WHEN FOOD IS YOUR DRUG

Most of us use food for comfort now and then. But some of us use food more like a drug. According to the National Association of Anorexia Nervosa and Associated Disorders, approximately seven million post-pubescent girls and women and one million post-pubescent boys and men in the United States struggle with eating disorders or borderline conditions.

Although I am not a certified counselor for eating disorders, I have made observations drawn from years of experience both as an eating-disorder survivor and as someone who has helped hundreds of women to form a healthy relationship with food. If you believe you have an eating disorder, I strongly urge you to seek medical supervision and address your emotional issues proactively. This chapter will offer additional help by illuminating the crucial chemical and nutritional factors that are too often overlooked in conventional treatment as well as the dubiously short-sighted approaches that typically take their place. But even if your relationship with food is relatively healthy or only mildly addictive, the insights that follow may help you resolve or avoid negative food issues altogether.

size has little to do with it

You don't need to have an eating disorder to get fat, and you certainly don't need to be fat to have an eating disorder. People often make the mistake of assuming otherwise, and even the medical world can overlook a person's eating disorder because that person is a normal size. Thin people with eating disorders can suffer terribly, thinking of food every minute and destroying their metabolisms by starving for days after a binge. This can be worse for your health than getting big by eating gradually.

are you addicted to food?

Here are ten signs—both mild and severe—that you may be using food as a drug:

- You need a sugar or caffeine fix to get you from lunch to dinner.
- You regularly reward yourself with large amounts of food and then feel guilt or shame.
- You feel the urge to binge when you are upset.
- You skip meals purposely and then gorge in one sitting.
- You get a buzz from food.
- You salivate over food advertisements.
- You prefer to eat alone so you can eat all you want in peace.
- You obsess about your next meal, even while full from the previous one.
- You worry about not getting enough food when you have to share.
- You continue to eat even after you experience physical discomfort from an overly full stomach.

the three ingredients of food obsession

When food is used as padding from our pain, our challenges, or a life we cannot fully embrace, it becomes a drug. And make no mistake: food—like drugs—can have strong chemical effects. It can produce a serotonin rush and can even cause the body to release natural opiates. In some cases, fermentation in the stomach can raise one's blood-alcohol level and cause an intoxicating effect similar to alcohol. I call this buzz the "elation and sedation effect." People aren't born with this chemical relationship with food; they develop it.

An addictive relationship with food requires three factors:

- The emotional need for the "drug" (food)
- The chemical relationship with food that lets you use it as a drug
- The drug-like foods themselves and their prevalence in your life

The combination of these three factors is the key to both the development of food obsession and complete freedom from it. Dealing with one aspect of the problem alone, such as emotional issues or better food choices, is never enough. Only when we orchestrate all three aspects at once will the demon finally flee. But too often the approach people take to deal with their food issues does not address any of these factors.

the eat-less/move-more approach leaves food obsession intact

People don't realize that those with eating disorders don't just deal with hunger but also with a chemical addiction triggered by emotional cues. Bingeing and starving are merely symptoms and side effects of those issues. The weight-loss professionals' rule of thumb, "Don't eat unless you're hungry," doesn't help someone with an eating problem, and it may actually prompt more starving, bingeing, and shame.

The clinical approach to eating disorders typically combines therapy and often antidepressants with nutritional counseling. It also entails learning about calories and fat grams and identifying the triggers behind emotional eating. Talking about your problems and exploring the emotional issues that make you use food as a drug is crucial. If you seek therapy, be sure to find an experienced counselor with a successful track record with eating disorders. If you get nutritional counseling, make sure that you see someone who is knowledgeable about the use of supplements to address the hormonal and mood issues (i.e., nutrient deficiencies and insulin, blood-sugar, thyroid, and serotonin inbalances). A successful program should make you feel supported and relieved and lead you to comfortable change. If something doesn't feel quite right, don't ignore the feeling. Try another counselor or get additional support elsewhere. Finally, whether you undergo counseling or not, remember that it ultimately comes down to you; don't fall into the trap of waiting for the answer from someone else.

EXERCISE CAUTION

Compulsion can thrive and express itself through strict dieting and exercise programs and must be dealt with separately from weight loss. If you feel ashamed of yourself or inadequate if you skip a workout, the overall effect is negative. Don't focus on exercise as the cure for your problem, and don't feel bad if it doesn't result in weight loss.

If you are addicted to food, don't let friends or doctors convince you that exercise can solve your problem or that your problem is due to lack of exercise. Once you've addressed your nutritional and chemical imbalances, you will begin to feel like moving again, and you will take joy in your body and the activity. Exercise that is properly fueled and performed harmoniously will have a positive impact on your biochemical balance and your mood.

starve your vice of its support through a process of shedding

Like other types of compulsive self-sabotage such as smoking and drinking, addiction to food is tricky to break free from because you not only have cultural and logistical influences to deal with but also the more complex conundrums of chemical and emotional issues that feed and perpetuate each other. But nothing can lead you more steadily toward freedom than the process of shedding, which systematically starves the emotional and chemical roots of the acts and substances that keep them alive and loosens their grip until they let go.

- *Give up the rules, the numbers, and the scale*. Preset menus and strict food lists encourage us to give up control and skip the thinking process. Creative calorie counting and weigh-ins put emphasis on numbers, which are deceiving and needlessly discouraging. All calories are not created equal, and neither are pounds. Forget calories and fat grams and the scale. Numbers are distractions from the real problem, and they cause more guilt-trips.

- *Uproot your emotional triggers and family legacies*. If you are able to uncover and reject anything that has been "bestowed" or projected upon you by a parent or a traumatic experience, you will begin to dispel the inexplicable shame that often propels a person toward self-sabotage. By going through this effort now you may also spare your own children the same legacy. Mother-daughter relationships, and sometimes father-daughter relationships, are behind most of the eating disorders and other self-destructive vices I see in the women who seek my help. Get some physical and emotional space.

- *Get angry, and then let it go*. Don't wait for apologies or answers from others who've done you wrong or contributed to your problem. Tell them exactly how you feel. Express your anger, but keep in mind that the worse this person treated you, the less likely you are to get an admission or an apology from him or her. Realize that by waiting for one, you could go on putting your life on hold forever. Move ahead. Only you can change your situation now.

- *Give yourself emotional padding to replace the physical and chemical padding that your vice provides*. Perfectionism and harsh self-judgment are usually a part of food obsession. They are signs that we are challenged in the area of unconditional self-love. Give yourself permission to fail at all of the what-ifs and the thin dreams that you've accumulated. This diffuses the power of a very deep-seated fear that your skinny best still won't be good enough. Unconditional self-love is the only padding that can replace the padding your vice gives you from your pain. Failure without an excuse is a scary prospect you never have to face as long as you have your weight problem as a buffer between you and your feelings and challenges.

don't settle for a weight-loss plan; strategize a health-gain plan

Don't call it a weight problem. Don't let even your doctor call it that anymore. Weight is just a symptom. Even if your doctor is focused on getting your weight into the "healthy" range, you can have more success and lose weight as a side effect if you set out to regain your *health* instead.

Plan a strategy to balance the health issues that affect you. Read up on every symptom and issue you have. If you go to a nutritionist, don't settle for calorie-focused information. Explore food sensitivities, metabolism, detoxification, and blood-sugar, thyroid, hormonal, and serotonin issues. Compulsion isn't something that average family doctors or nutritionists should take on unless it is their area of specialty. And even if you do find someone who specializes in eating disorders, make sure you continue exploring cutting-edge nutrition and alternative therapies.

MOLLY AND FEN-PHEN

Several years ago, I did the makeup for a model named Molly, who told me that she hadn't been able to keep any food down, except a bit here and there, for days. At the advice of her agent, she had been taking the popular but controversial weight-loss drug Fenfluramine-Phentermine (Fen-phen).

The woman was extremely skinny, even for a model, so it blew my mind that someone with a medical license would give her this drug, which even then—before it was found to be deadly—was to be prescribed only to the substantially overweight. As Molly walked onto the set, she told me that she had temporarily lost her sight just a few days before and that the doctor had given her another drug to counteract that side effect. As I watched her pose, I actually saw her sway. It was amazing that this stranger had just told me this without blinking an eye. She was clearly calling out for help she wasn't getting elsewhere. In between shots, I gave her a special "meal cookie" I had made at home with nuts, flaxseeds, pumpkinseeds, grated carrots, and soy flour. Later in the day she told me that this was the first food that had stayed down in days. When we finished the shoot, I gave her the number of an alternative doctor in Manhattan experienced with weaning people off Fen-phen.

Molly left the job before I could get her number, so at a chance meeting a few years later I was happy to see she was doing well. She expressed deep gratitude for my referral to the doctor who had led her to freedom from Fen-phen. From the short time she was on the drug, she had already suffered some permanent effects that require her to take precautions, such as taking antibiotics when having her teeth cleaned, but she is alive and well.

This poem offers perhaps the best example I've come across of how to give ourselves the emotional "padding" and sanctuary of unconditional self-love. At the same time, it illustrates the courage it takes to let ourselves be uncovered and to give up the protective "layers" that obscure our inner beauty. The author is unknown.

The Difference Between Strength and Courage

It takes strength to be firm,

It takes courage to be gentle,

It takes strength to stand guard,

It takes courage to let down your guard,

It takes strength to conquer,

It takes courage to surrender,

It takes strength to be certain,

It takes courage to have doubt,

It takes strength to fit in,

It takes courage to stand out,

It takes strength to feel a friend's pain,

It takes courage to feel your own pain,

It takes strength to hide your own pains,

It takes courage to show them,

It takes strength to endure abuse,

It takes courage to stop it,

It takes strength to stand alone,

It takes courage to lean on another,

It takes strength to love,

It takes courage to be loved,

It takes strength to survive,

It takes courage to live.

it's never all in your head

Finally, you must remember that whether your vice is drinking, smoking, or eating, there are chemical reasons behind it all.

Millions of people face sugar and carb addictions to varying degrees—particularly in the aftermath of the fat-free era. For many it will take more than attempted abstinence from carbs to escape their grip. If you are addicted to carbs, they will be your drug until you no longer have a hypersensitive chemical relationship with them and you no longer need to be drugged to deal with your emotions.

Whether you are the average person who struggles with carb cravings or someone with an eating disorder, there remains one great barrier to the higher-protein, lower-glycemic answer: the prevalence, convenience, and addictive nature of refined carbs. It's unlikely that conventional medicine and clinical nutrition will soon endorse the healthiest, easiest, drug-free escape from that merry-go-round: unpatentable, natural supplements.

Before you embark on the next attempt to change your relationship with food, be sure to give yourself every advantage and support.

STACY: ANATOMY OF A TOTAL TRANSFORMATION

"If they only knew" was what I thought as I looked at my co-workers. I am highly respected at my marketing firm. My co-workers saw a "together" woman of relatively normal weight who they knew was a freak about the "F word" (fat). Little did they know that once alone at home, I had this freakish life of torment with food. In order to protect myself from my own inevitable nightly binges, I stocked up on my special foods that allowed me to binge with minimal repercussions. Each night featured the same ludicrous scene: I'd go in and out of the kitchen, battling the gravitational pull to the box of Luna bars or the half-gallon of fat-free ice cream. "No, I should go to sleep! Am I going to do it? No . . . Yes." This was my secret hell.

I had already been to a nutritionist, who got me eating much healthier food in general. I thought it would help, but to my surprise, it had little effect on my secret problem. I began to wonder if my own emotional issues were worse than I wanted to admit. I had binged and gone through stages of purging through college, but I had figured out how to binge on completely empty foods and minimize the weight gain. My life was not my own, and I didn't sleep. My body was agitated and I was truly obsessed with food.

My nutritionist got me to attend Kat's program, and after seeing her own history and transformation and knowing she could truly relate, I was finally convinced not only to try to eat some fat but also to take supplements to help my cravings and moods. I started eating plain, regular, organic yogurt and berries for breakfast (instead of artificially sweetened, nonfat yogurt); drinking green tea and a great-tasting herbal coffee you brew in the coffeemaker (tastes the same—only better) instead of coffee. I started making Kat's decadent salads for lunch, adding garnishes I would *never* have touched before, like nuts, cheese, and olive oil, and taking essential fatty acids, chromium, 5HTP, carb blockers, and melatonin at night. During the first couple of days, I tried one of Kat's tricks at a staff meeting where there were only bagels and cream cheese to eat. My co-workers' jaws dropped and even I was having an out-of-body experience when I took half a bagel and piled on some cream cheese so I could eat it without starting my sugar pendulum. My co-workers had never seen me eat fat. After eating it, I felt calm and free of thoughts of food, cravings, and energy slumps until lunch, while everyone else kept making trips back to the pastry tray. At lunch, one woman in the office was entranced by the arugula salad I was eating at my desk. People have a powerful response when they see real, beautifully prepared food in a setting where we so often abuse ourselves.

It has been only one month since I made these changes, and my bingeing has stopped. I don't remember when it fully stopped, but for the last couple of weeks, I have been able to sit alone in my own house and—incredibly—not have obsessive thoughts or feel that menacing pull toward the refrigerator. Those nights feel like a distant memory, though it was such a short time ago. And since I started taking melatonin and using a sleep mask, I have been sleeping through the night until my alarm goes off, which is also a first. And the sleep, along with my sane relationship with food, has really changed something in me. I have always been a confident woman and I have loved my career, but for the first time in so long, I am feeling "pretty."

I have emotional issues like everyone else, but they are much less of a factor than I had thought. Something in my head has clicked in a big way. It has affected my attitude toward myself and my definition of food, but it is more a result of what has happened than the cause. I am free of the real cause of the craziness, and I know exactly what it was now. There is no struggle and no desire to go back. I have learned to free myself.

It's impossible to predict the day your demon will let go, but it will if you continue to shed the layers of issues that feed it. When it does, it will be merely a thrilling side effect of a much more profound transformation you have already begun.

Chapter 8

ACHIEVE MAXIMUM RADIANCE WITH SUPPLEMENTS

"The fruit thereof shall be your meat,
and the leaf your medicine."
—Ezekiel 47:12

It's hard for me to contain my enthusiasm for supplements. As an informed layperson who saved my own health and transformed my appearance with their crucial help, I consider supplements a key component of any serious beauty and body arsenal. Changing my head may have been crucial to overcoming my eating disorder, but using supplements to change my *chemical* relationship with food is what truly freed me from food addiction and healed the other serious health issues and imbalances caused by over a decade of self-abuse. I give supplements full credit for reversing my liver disorder and many other issues I'd been told I would be stuck with for the rest of my life.

But maybe you take far better care of yourself than I once did, which is quite likely. Is it possible that you have sidestepped the need for supplements by doing all the right things? Are healthier food choices, exercise, and stress management enough to protect your precious vitality? Take this quiz and find out.

Which statement applies to you?

- I don't drink coffee, alcohol, or smoke.
- I eat only organic foods.
- I don't live in a polluted environment.
- I am not currently taking any prescription drugs.
- I don't drink or shower in chlorinated water.
- I have never taken antibiotics.
- I eat primarily raw, locally grown, organic food.
- I juice at least once a week.
- I am not under a lot of stress.

If all of the above apply to you, you might not need to take supplements, but it still wouldn't hurt.

Keep in mind that though vitamins and minerals are naturally occurring substances, they are also chemicals that can interact and compete with other substances in your bloodstream. Always read and ask your healthcare provider about your particular health concerns and the supplements you take and how they might react with prescription medications you may be using. Because such information can be hard to find, I've provided a list in the Resources of some of the best sources that even your doctor will respect and understand, like the *Physician's Desk Reference Herbal*.

While far fewer double-blind clinical trials are conducted on natural (unpatentable) substances than on synthetic drugs, much of the evidence supporting the supplements covered in the following pages is more conclusive than the conflicting science behind conventional controversies, such as mammograms, the role of dietary cholesterol in heart disease, low-fat diets, and certain surgical procedures. If supplements such EFAs were

> **MYTH: *There's no need to supplement if I eat well.***
>
> **TRUTH: *Healthy foods aren't what they used to be.***
>
> We've been told all our lives that eating a well-balanced diet with plenty of fruits and vegetables will keep us well nourished. But how many of us are eating the recommended nine servings? Even if we were, all those fruits and vegetables are unlikely to provide adequate nourishment. Although it has not been widely publicized, U.S. and Canadian food tables show declining nutrient levels in conventionally grown produce due to depleted minerals in the soil. More food nutrients are lost through processing, transport time, storage, and cooking methods. We may eat perfectly, but we still have to live in an imperfect world.

patentable synthetic drugs, the million-dollar commercial might go something like this: "Common side effects include relief from dry skin; silkier hair; anti-inflammatory effects throughout the body; reduced joint pain; improved immunity, hormone function, moods, and cholesterol levels; and countless other desirables. Warning: Nature heals in ways we can only begin to predict."

nature in therapeutic doses

No conventional doctor has ever warned me of the dangers of eating depleted foods. They tend to focus only on calorie intake. And if they are unconcerned with the harm and gradual malnourishment that comes from eating empty foods, it isn't really a surprise that they don't seem to care about the importance of putting those nutrients back. If you don't look into what quality supplements can do for you, you are short-changing nature's intention for you by denying yourself the most intuitive, therapeutic way to replenish yourself in this depleted and denatured world.

MYTH: **Dietary supplements are unregulated and unproven.**

TRUTH: **Dietary supplements are regulated under the 1994 Dietary Supplement Health Education Act (DSHEA).**

The next time people tell you that supplements are unregulated, set them straight. Supplements are subject to extensive labeling requirements, including full disclosure of ingredients, nutrition information, and censorship of health-benefit claims by the FDA. Many leading experts in the fields of complementary and alternative medicine believe that health claims for supplements are unfairly suppressed, despite the increasing amount of scientific evidence showing their benefits, such as protection against certain cancers, reversal of dysplasia (abnormal cell growth), lowered cholesterol, decreased inflammation, relief from depression, improved insulin action, birth-defect prevention, and bone-loss prevention.

Just about every nutrient has an effect on how you look and feel. As to whether the benefits of supplements are proven, according to Dr. Julian Whitaker, director of the Whitaker Wellness Institute and editor of the newsletter *Health and Healing*, more than eight thousand clinical studies attest to the protective effects of individual antioxidant vitamins, minerals, and extracts from mushrooms, herbs, and other medicinal plants.

get gorgeous by guarding your health

Because beauty and health are inseparable, it's impossible to improve one area without experiencing good side effects in the other. What might be the best regimens for health issues like breast-cancer prevention are also some of the best supplements for your skin and your body. For example, alpha-lipoic acid detoxifies the body, recycles antioxidants for anti-aging and beautiful skin, and helps stabilize blood sugar for a beautiful body. Both green tea and selenium have been shown to help prevent skin and breast cancer. Tocotrienols, a category of vitamin E components that inhibits human breast-cancer cell lines in culture, are now believed to offer possibly greater antioxidant protection to the skin than the traditional, well-studied alpha-tocopherol form of vitamin E. Dr. Nicholas Perricone notes that tocotrienols reduce redness and flaking in severely dry skin, prevent nails from cracking, and even make the hair shinier.

HOW CARMEN CONQUERED HER VARICOSE VEINS AND BECAME A CONVERT

Carmen, a bus driver who consulted with me in New York, got excited when I told her about the studies that showed horse-chestnut-seed extract could shrink the swelling of varicose veins as well as compression-hose therapy and could actually decrease ankle circumference in women with varicose veins (chronic venous insufficiency)—all this while improving vascular function throughout the entire body.

Carmen was so amazed and inspired by the improvement in her varicose veins after only a few weeks of using horse-chestnut-seed extract that she decided to start taking other supplements, like essential fatty acids, quercetin, nettle, and methylsulfonylmethane (MSM). She soon noticed an improvement in her allergies and psoriasis. Her skin no longer burned in the shower and she was able to sit outside at her sister's country home in upstate New York for the first time without having an allergy attack. "I feel like these supplements have taken ten years off of my life," said Carmen.

Did you know that

- A six-month regimen of folic acid, vitamin B12, and vitamin B6 can help prevent recurrence of blocked arteries in patients who have undergone coronary angioplasty.

- Chromium picolinate has been proven in multiple human studies to build muscle while eliminating fat, improve cholesterol levels, stabilize blood sugar, and even reverse certain types of diabetes. Because of its ability to lower and control blood-sugar levels, chromium is considered a valuable tool against glycosylation, or protein degradation caused by sugar, which can rapidly age the body and the skin.

- Selenium reduced cancer mortality in humans by 50 percent over ten years in a study published in the Journal of the American Medical Association.

- Hydroxycitric acid, an extract from the plant *Garcinia cambogia*, both curbs your appetite and blocks the synthesis of body fat.

- Taking calcium-containing antacid neutralizes stomach acid, making its calcium unabsorbable.

- Essential fatty acids (EFAs) actually help release fat from the body in addition to maintaining so many health factors which affect your quality of life that they could almost be considered a panacea. Hormone balance, cholesterol ratios, skin and hair health, joint flexibility, moods, and immunity have all been proven to be helped by EFAs.

- The ingredients of a calcium supplement called AdvaCal have been shown in clinical research to actually increase bone density.

anti-aging supplements: fact or fiction?

Scientific panels are still debating whether supplements contain anti-aging attributes. The conservative, traditional position has been that they do not; however, compelling research, including an animal study that showed a clear reversal of age-related memory, mobility, and cellular decline in rats from a combination of alpha-lipoic acid and acetyl L-carnitine, strongly supports the contrary.

Many people are familiar with the aging effects of free radicals, the harmful compounds generated in our bodies by sun exposure, smoking, unhealthy foods, and other lifestyle assaults. Free radicals contribute to degenerative diseases and to the dreaded collagen cross-linking that causes wrinkles. New science points to another basic cause of aging: glycation, a sugar-related "browning" process that degrades proteins and turns them into advanced glycation end products (AGEs). As AGEs accumulate throughout the body, they generate more compounded free radicals and cross-linking on their own, causing a domino effect.

Perhaps one of the most exciting supplements in the anti-aging arena is the substance carnosine (not to be confused with L-carnitine). Animal studies have shown it inhibits the glycation process. In fact, one study showed that carnosine not only extended lifespan and improved brain function but that it actually also improved the appearance of tested rats by keeping fur dark and glossy and reducing skin ulcers.

The hormones DHEA and hGH—both native to the body—have also been proven to reverse signs of aging in humans when augmented by supplementation or injection, respectively. The latter can have side effects and should be approached cautiously, but according to Oz Garcia, author of *Look and Feel Fabulous Forever*, there are well over two thousand published studies demonstrating DHEA's ability to improve age-related stress, immune, hormonal, weight, and heart issues. Garcia suggests taking salivary or blood tests under medical supervision to monitor any hormone treatments.

ANOTHER BEAUTIFUL REASON TO QUIT SMOKING

In October 2002, scientists at the Scripps Research Institute in La Jolla, California, announced that smoking accelerates the glycation process. A nicotine by-product caused an accelerated "cooking" of proteins and formation of health- and skin-destroying AGEs. This discovery should provide yet another incentive for smokers concerned with both beauty as well as health to kick the habit.

regimens of the future: genetics and nutrition work together

Science has revealed that it's not necessarily your genes that determine the fate of your health but rather if and when those genes are expressed. In some cases, nutritional strategies can play a role in minimizing that expression. In the August 2002 edition of *Health and Healing*, Dr. Julian Whitaker stated that someone with a family history of colon cancer can reduce the doubled risk of getting colon cancer to that of the average person by taking 400 mcg of folic acid every day. Similarly, people born with an inability to convert omega-6 fatty acids to the anti-inflammatory gamma linoleic (GLA) form may be more likely to have eczema, but GLA supplementation is believed to somewhat make up for this deficiency and its symptoms, such as itching, flaking, inflammation, and dryness. In a letter published in the *New England Journal of Medicine*, Robert M. Hoover, M.D., of the National Cancer Institute wrote that "genes and environment interact to produce a risk greater than the sum of their independent effects."

start with a high-quality, high-potency vitamin regimen

All vitamins are not created equal. You get what you pay for. Avoid little pills that have 100 percent of all the Recommended Dietary Allowances (RDAs). They're useless. One little pill cannot give you everything you need. And in order to be absorbed by your body, you need more food-like forms of nutrients that require bulk. It's not just what you take but also what your body absorbs that counts.

RDAs are dated recommendations that were developed to prevent malnutrition or deficiencies, not to promote optimal health. The most advanced full-spectrum multi-nutrient regimens contain therapeutically proven potencies of nutrients that far exceed RDAs. They often look like horse pills or consist of multiple capsules and oil pills (EFAs don't combine well in pills or capsules), have a distinctive odor when fresh (if a tablet), and are usually taken three times a day (although one of these pills would likely give you more benefit than a week's worth of once-a-day little pills). Any worthwhile full-spectrum multi-nutrient formula will set you back about forty or more dollars for a month's supply, but they will likely save you untold doctor bills, sick days, and lost vitality and beauty in the long run.

You'll find quality multi-nutrient regimens at good health-food or vitamin stores and on-line. See the Resources for some of the best multi-nutrient regimens.

Signs of Quality

- Avoid the cheapest vitamins, generic drugstore brands, and brands filled with di-calcium phosphate, cellulose, and other fillers. United States Pharmacopeia (USP) vitamins are all synthetic. A handful of studies show decreased absorption or benefit in certain synthetic vitamins, such as dl-alpha tocopherol (the synthetic form of vitamin E), while the d-alpha natural form was more beneficial. Isolated vitamins may not be as absorbable by the body as natural, or food-based, vitamins, although many quality products incorporate both.

- Look for mixed carotenoids. Recent studies show that mixed carotenoids—not just beta-carotene by itself—work together to protect the skin against the harmful effects of ultraviolet radiation and reduce DNA damage, one of the leading causes of many types of cancer.

- Look for mixed tocopherols rather than just alpha-tocopherol (vitamin E) and bioflavanoids like quercetin rather than just vitamin C. Look for the more absorbable calcium citrate over calcium carbonate. Look for turmeric and green tea; phytochemicals like ellagic acid, lycopene, and lutein; and super-foods like chlorella.

basic supplements with beauty side effects

The nutritional supplements listed in the charts that follow are some of the most well-researched and highly regarded in the field at this writing. Amazingly, each of these all-star supplements initiates a chain reaction of improvements that will almost certainly have effects on beauty issues and shape as well as health. My goal is to get you excited about the incredible quality of life and vitality to be gained from supplements and to provide the most user-friendly resources so you can make your own discoveries and bring them to the attention of your healthcare provider when appropriate. Most of these supplements are available at vitamin stores. Ordering information for hard-to-find products is listed in the Resources.

The information in this chapter, as in the others, is not intended to diagnose or treat disease. Enlist your doctor's supervision when treating health issues with supplements. For medical references and more information, visit the Life Extension Foundation's Web site, www.lef.org.

Nutrient	Benefit
High-potency multivitamin and minerals regimens	Benefits range from lowered risk of heart disease and stroke to prevention of birth defects and everything in between. **Beauty side effects:** Vary according to formula, but the first change a person usually notices is decreased cravings and increased energy.
Green powder *Includes barley grass, spirulina, and wheat grass.*	Green powders are full of enzymes, phytochemicals, and body-detoxifying chlorophyll. **Beauty side effects:** Beautiful, clear skin; faster healing of bruises due to enzymes and vitamin K.
EFAs *Includes flax, borage, evening primrose, and fish oils.*	EFAs have cardiovascular and antidepressant effects. **Beauty side effects:** Anti-inflammatory; replenishes healing lipids to the skin and hair.
Probiotics *Includes acidophilus and other strains of beneficial bacteria.*	Rebalances the good bacteria in the gut for better digestion and immunity. **Beauty side effects:** Improved digestion clears the skin and diminishes sensitivity and some inflammatory skin conditions.
Vitamin C *Buy vitamin C with bioflavanoids for greater benefits.*	Boosts immunity, heart protection, and fights free radicals. **Beauty side effects:** Boosts collagen formation and the skin's natural protection from sun damage.

Continued on the next page

Nutrient	Benefit
N-acetyl cysteine (NAC)	NAC forms glutathione, a key detoxifying agent in the body. Many doctors consider glutathione to be the body's primary protection against cellular damage. **Beauty side effects:** Increased detoxification clears the skin.
Alpha-lipoic acid	Lipoic acid, the universal antioxidant, recycles other antioxidants in the body and scavenges more types of free radicals than any other known antioxidant. **Beauty side effects:** Antioxidant, anti-aging, and anti-inflammatory for the skin.
Siberian ginseng	Protects the adrenals from exhaustion caused by chronic stress. Adrenals that work better can protect the body from chronically elevated cortisol levels, which can in turn wreak havoc on bones and cause fat accumulation. **Beauty side effects:** Improved adrenal function, which diminishes allergies, under-eye circles, and puffiness in the face and body; decreased stress reaction in skin and stomach fat due to excess cortisol.
Coenzyme Q10 (CoQ10) *Always buy oil-based capsules for better absorption.*	A powerful anti-aging, free radical–scavenging, and proven breast cancer– and heart disease–inhibiting enzyme. Be sure to buy the oil-based gelcap for better absorption. Note that this important cellular rejuvenator is depleted by cholesterol-lowering drugs. **Beauty side effects:** Increases cellular energy and may stimulate tissue regeneration. As a powerful antioxidant it may fight photo-aging and environmental skin effects.
Vitamin E *Buy the natural form for proven increased effectiveness. You'll get maximum benefit from mixed tocopherol forms, which include gamma tocopherol.*	Benefits the cardiovascular system. **Beauty side effects:** Antioxidant and environmental skin protection.

Nutrient	Benefit
Carnosine *Note: Not to be confused with the amino acid L-carnitine (below).*	This anti-aging substance has been found to extend lifespan, inhibit glycation throughout the body, and reverse the physical changes and mental decline associated with aging in rats. **Beauty side effects:** May inhibit skin and body aging from glycation.
L-carnitine, or Acetyl L-carnitine	Heart-protective, blood sugar–stabilizing supplement. **Beauty side effects:** In combination with alpha-lipoic acid, it has been shown to reverse many effects of aging. It also helps weight loss.

supplements that help balance weight-related health issues

A variety of hormonal and chemical factors you may not even have considered may be dominating your body and keeping you from losing weight.

The following supplements not only helped me change my chemical relationship with food but actually re-proportioned my body from "pear" to normal and helped me regain my health in many other ways in the process.

But don't run out and buy them all! First identify your issues with your doctor and zero in on the support you need. If you are currently taking or considering prescription weight-loss drugs, ask your doctor if any of these alternatives could spare you the possible side effects, such as the kidney and liver concerns associated with Meridia (sibutramine hydrochloride monohydrate) or the incontinence risks of Xenical (Orlistat).

Weight-Related Issues	Proven Supplement Support
Blood sugar and cravings	• Chromium (polynicotinate form might have advantages over picolinate) • Alpha-lipoic acid • Vanadyl sulfate • *Garcinia cambogia* (Citrimax) • Gymnema sylvestre
Mood, stress, and anxiety	• Relora: More research is needed, but preliminary studies suggest that it decreases cortisol levels which can contribute to fat accumulation in the midsection. It induces relaxation and increases DHEA levels. • 5-HTP has been shown to increase serotonin levels and reduce anxiety without side effects.
Fat metabolism/absorption	• Hydroxycitric acid, a rare fruit acid from the Garcinia cambogia fruit, has been shown in numerous studies to increase thermogenesis (calorie burning), prevent fat storage, and reduce appetite. • Green tea • CLA • MCT oil • Choline • Inositol • L-methionine • Chitosan is shellfish cartilage that absorbs fat. Liquid chitosan (FTF) is the only form I'm aware of that doesn't cause any digestive problems. Chitosan absorbs healthy fat, so you shouldn't take it when eating healthy fats or with your vitamins.
Carbohydrate metabolism *Take these supplements one-half hour before meals.*	Carb blockers such as Carb Cutter, Carb Slasher, and other Phaseolamin-containing supplements block the enzymes that digest carbs. They really help to get you off the sugar pendulum and make a difference you can feel after the first time you use them.

Weight-Related Issues	Proven Supplement Support
Hormones balancers and releasers *These supplements are not hormones themselves. Natural hormones like DHEA can have amazing beauty and quality-of-life benefits but should be used with close doctor supervision.*	• Chaste tree berry (vitex) has demonstrated the unique ability to subtly and safely balance estrogen and progesterone levels that can help normalize weight. • Kelp and L-tyrosine stoke a sluggish thyroid. • The amino acids L-ornithine and L-arginine help you release hGH, which keeps you lean.

HOW KELLY LOST THE FINAL TEN

When I consulted with Kelly, a petite woman at 5'2", about her weight, energy, and food issues, I found that she was already eating quality, fresh, real food that she prepared daily from scratch. But Kelly had major issues with energy that required her to take an afternoon nap to get through the day. I encouraged Kelly to look into supplements and how they might increase her energy and address her energy dips. She was skeptical, but after looking at some compelling scientific research, Kelly began taking an advanced multi-nutrient regimen. After a couple months, she added a supplement that combined CoQ10 and the amino acid L-carnitine to her regimen after reading about their proven energizing and heart-health effects. Soon Kelly's reservations about the efficacy of supplements were eliminated. She was amazed to find herself skipping her usual nap and staying productive throughout the day. Even more surprising, Kelly lost just over ten pounds over the next couple of months. "That's major," she said. "I've been trying to lose that final ten for nearly a decade." And when she stopped taking the multivitamin regimen after running out, her appetite and cravings returned. That's how much our body needs nutrients we so often deprive it of.

pro-beauty probiotics: feed your good bugs

Our modern lifestyle poses a challenge to the good bacteria (probiotics) that dwell in our guts. From the drugs we take to the chlorinated water we drink and shower in, our precious bugs are fighting for survival. And when they start to lose, more virulent bad bugs, like the *Candida albicans* strain, can rule over our gut and other parts of our bodies. This can contribute to a stubborn imbalance of good and bad bacteria and yeast in the gut and even on the skin, which can set the stage for myriad autoimmune syndromes and "skindromes."

Consuming probiotics and taking other steps to regain your pro-beauty ecology may help with a range of problems, including acne, poor digestion, itchy skin, dandruff, athlete's foot, allergies, and sinus and vaginal yeast issues. These factors are merely symptoms of a more serious syndrome that often includes autoimmune diseases, nutritional deficiencies, and food sensitivities.

The Simple Solutions

- Take a good probiotic, which you'll find at a quality vitamin store.
- Eat a lot of plain yogurt and drink kefir (always unsweetened).
- Starve your yeast of the sugar, flour, and starch on which it thrives.
- Eat loads of garlic, which kills yeast and just about any other bacteria.
- Take a yeast-fighting supplement, such as Candex.
- Install water and shower filters to minimize chlorine, which can contribute to probiotic depletion in the body.

protect your breasts as you beautify your skin and detoxify your body

Certain toxins in our environment, water, and skin products have now been shown to accumulate in breast tissue and breast milk. I see breasts as two small (or voluptuous) microcosms of the world we live in. Rejuvenate your entire body and your peace of mind by eating and supplementing for your breasts.

What protects the breasts also creates beautiful skin and a healthy body. For example, omega-3 fatty acids from fish oil may offer protection from breast cancer and benign breast disease. At the same time they may help relieve eczema. Chlorella has been shown to bind with heavy metals and pesticides and remove them from the body, to detoxify carcinogenic substances, and also to help heal skin wounds.

Breast Supplement Superstars	Benefit
D-glucarate (in broccoli)	D-glucarate has been shown to inhibit proliferative estrogens and breast-tumor formation.
Indole-3 carbinol (from cruciferous vegetables)	I3C from cabbage inhibited growth of estrogen receptor-positive breast-cancer cells better than tamoxifen in one study.
Green tea	Green tea increases the body's key detoxifying substance, glutathione. It has been shown to cause apoptosis, or cancer-cell death.
Curcumin (in turmeric)	In addition to being an antioxidant and anti-inflammatory, curcumin has also been shown to block harmful estrogen-mimicking chemicals.
Milk thistle/Silibinin	Milk thistle detoxifies and regenerates liver tissue and has been shown to inhibit cancer cell replication and to make some types of chemotherapy more effective.
Melatonin	An association between decreased melatonin levels and breast-cancer risk has been suggested and is being further investigated with regard to sun and sleep factors. Lower levels of melatonin have been linked with eating disorders and insulin resistance.
Tocotrienols	Tocotrienols from palm oil demonstrated anti-proliferative effects on human breast-cancer cell lines. Dr. Perricone recommends them for beautiful skin.

DETOXIFICATION AND GLUTATHIONE

Many pioneers in nutritional research believe that glutathione levels in the body are key to how well we detoxify the endless chemicals and heavy metals we are exposed to. Glutathione is found in cruciferous vegetables and garlic. Supplementation with N-acetylcysteine (NAC) has been shown to raise blood-glutathione levels significantly.

CAN GOING "WIRELESS" KEEP BREASTS HEALTHIER?

In 1996, an unpublished study of 4,700 women supported what some doctors have suggested in the past, only to encounter mockery: Bras are unhealthy for breasts. In the study, those who wore a bra twenty-four hours a day had breast-cancer rates 125 times higher than those who wore no bra at all. The scientists theorize that bras restrict lymph drainage in the breast area, which allows toxins to build. Bear in mind that this study did not factor in lifestyle conditions or use controls and was not published in a respected medical journal. In the meantime, consider a bra that doesn't bind or constrict.

supplement sense

Start slow. Introduce only a couple of vitamins and only one herb at a time unless otherwise directed by your healthcare provider. And, as always, stay informed. Supplements are natural substances that may still cause reactions and side effects, although rare. It's your responsibility to find out what those may be before putting them into your body.

Comprehensive information on any dangers or possible interactions between supplements and drugs can be found in references such as the *Physician's Desk Reference Herbal* and other such books (see the Resources). Tell your doctor what you're planning to take, particularly if you are getting other forms of traditional healthcare, and get hooked up to a steady stream of information so you can continue to expand your knowledge and options.

making supplements an autopilot beauty ritual

Remember to start with a quality full-spectrum multivitamin and mineral regimen. I've listed several that deliver therapeutic potencies in the Resources. But don't go overboard. Be aware that combining nutrition bars, fortified foods, and meal-replacement shakes can give you too much of some nutrients, like vitamin A and iron, which can build up in the body. As you learn more, you can work with your doctor to tailor what you take to suit your particular health needs and your budget.

The keys to supplements are quality and consistency. The increasing availability of creams, sprays, and particularly patches that deliver supplements transdermally will make their use even more convenient and effective in the near future. With no more discipline than it takes to brush your teeth, you can experience physical and cellular transformation year after year. Many people have experienced the best health and looks of their life after forty because of the miracle of nature in therapeutic doses.

Part III

THE MAKEUP-LESS MAKEOVER

Chapter 9

GET BACK YOUR "VIRGIN" SKIN

To go without makeup is every woman's right. To look great without it is every woman's possibility. The most beautiful skin is supple, glowing, and hydrated and shows healthy circulation. And contrary to popular belief, even "perfect" skin bears the occasional, if not frequent, blemish. We can have perfect skin, but we still have to live in an imperfect world.

As someone who's been in contact with a new face—and heard a new skin story—just about every day since my beauty career began, I can often guess what a woman has been up to by looking closely at her face or at her hair. Interestingly, more and more of the skin problems I see are caused by the very regimens and treatments women use to make their skin beautiful. The tough surface, immovable blemishes, and oily rebound due to drying regimens; the rawness from overzealous lunchtime peels; the crepey, dry tightness of alpha hydroxy acid abuse or certain vitamin A–derivative treatments; the flaky patches caused by benzoyl peroxide dabbing—none of it wears makeup well. The concept of "normal" doesn't have much use in skin regimens anymore. Just about everyone's skin has been rendered somewhat sensitive by today's aggressive products and treatments.

beautiful skin shouldn't be hard work

Good skin isn't about doing a three-part regimen twice a day or keeping your face sterile and oil-free. It's about wisdom, strategy, and restraint. The idea that you're not doing enough of this or that is nonsense. More often than not it's what you *don't* do that makes your skin beautiful.

Healthy skin in a balanced body maintains itself with minimal fuss, renews itself at just the right pace, and glows on its own. In order to get to this point, you need to recover your skin's full, protective functions. If your skin is already healthy, this chapter will help you avoid the pitfalls that often jeopardize good skin. But if you have found yourself dependent on a skin regimen that has left your skin more sensitive or problematic, this is the road back to "virgin" skin. These are the first steps toward a truly holistic approach to your best skin ever.

peel back the layers of regimen overkill

Marketing mania has most of us convinced that nature in action is an unruly phenomenon to be neutralized or tamed. Advertisements teach us that hair follicles, sweat glands, surface-level skin cells, sebum, and all bacteria are beauty's mortal enemies. We are seduced into seeking the latest, harshest ways to show our hair, skin, and bodily functions who's in charge. We think nothing of using products that strip us of "bad" oil and peel away that "bad" surface skin because our poor bodies aren't as smart as the scientists who devise these approaches. We dab on blemish creams that kill all that "bad" bacteria while drying the skin into a drawn, lifeless state that is far removed from nature's intention. Real beauty has nothing to do with tingling, deep-cleaning, super-exfoliating products. These measures are overkill, and the costs to your skin, your hair, and possibly even your health can be considerable. Most of the new-and-improved (read: harsh) products and more aggressive exfoliating techniques compromise our skin's precious self-protective matrix. All of this has created a whole spectrum of new "skindromes" with equally unnatural new maintenance requirements. Before we know it, we're a slave to new skin problems and the upkeep these regimens create as we sacrifice the inherent self-protective potential as well as the natural glow our skin once had. These harsh approaches to skin care are based on the false assumption that our skin doesn't already come equipped with its own superior antibacterial, antiwrinkle, and anti-invader protection system.

treatment-caused "skindromes"

Certain skin products and regimens pose subtle, or sometimes major, irritations to the skin that compromise its ability to deal optimally with daily challenges. Just as your body must recover its original immunity after you eat sugar, your skin must recover its immunity after you treat your face with harsh detergents or toxic products. Some of us put a great deal of money and effort into fixing our skin without addressing the irritants that may be causing it to be vulnerable and reactive in the first place.

Common dermatological skin treatments can cause compounded problems that often make the original skin issue look like a walk in the park. One course of antibiotics for acne, for example, can destroy most of the protective bacteria that keep your gut in working order, leaving you with problems that are no longer skin-deep. Next thing you know, you could be suffering from yeast infections, malabsorption, food sensitivities, and a host of other problems, not to mention a wicked relapse of the original skin problem. Recurrences are especially likely if you use topical hydrocortisone ointments, which eventually thins the skin and wears down its natural immunity.

WEANING OFF OF STEROID CREAMS

Kathy received a consultation with me as a gift from her boyfriend. She had been struggling with a rash on her chin and using over-the-counter hydrocortisone ointment on it for almost a year. It always worked initially, but then the rash returned. She noticed that the patch of skin became increasingly crepey and translucent between outbreaks. When I told Kathy that steroid ointments thin the skin over time, she became interested in exploring alternatives. She was surprised that I began with a checklist of harmful habits to shed rather than leading her right to another product to replace the steroid ointment. No new cream was going to help as long as she was stripping and smothering her skin with irritating foaming cleansers and perfumed moisturizers and aggravating her skin with sugary, pro-inflammatory foods and drinks.

I advised Kathy to get a checkup to screen the prescription drugs she was taking for their possible effects on her skin and to pinpoint any other health issues signaled by her rashes. No matter what cream I suggested (licorice, chamomile, or pyrithione zinc–based products, in this case), she would have to go through steroid withdrawal and let the rash run its course at least once before it would begin to subside and the skin could recover its immunity.

In the meantime, she could greatly reduce inflammation and allergic responses by eliminating foods she was sensitive to and by using anti-inflammatory and immune-calming supplements. I gave Kathy abstracts from peer-reviewed studies on some of these substances so she could involve (and inform) her dermatologist and make her final choices with him. Finally, I introduced her to cosmetics that could cover the redness on her face without irritating her skin. It was clear at the end of our consultation that she was blown away that no one had ever told her she was destroying her skin's future with the steroid cream.

A couple of months later, Kathy told me she had not only stayed off the steroid cream but also her rash was finally gone and the redness that remained was subsiding. In addition, the supplements and the food and skin-product upgrades had dramatically changed her entire complexion as well as other issues. She felt better all over. And most exciting for me, she was thinking about quitting smoking, an area she would not negotiate at our initial consultation.

recover your skin's basic pro-beauty functions

Many of my past and present clients have applied a "first do no harm" philosophy to their skin issues and have been able to reverse the domino effect of skin regimens that were sensitizing and disabling their skin, wean themselves off of steroid creams and antibiotics, and even drastically change—or discover—their true skin type. Chances are your own skin problems are not entirely nature's doing, and the solution for them probably isn't something you can apply to the surface. In fact, it might be what you *stop* applying that has the greatest impact.

Like the rest of our bodies, our skin needs a sanctuary from irritants and assaults in order to recover its pro-beauty functions and reverse the compounded problems that can get out of control once these basic functions are compromised. In order to get back our virgin skin, we must

- Recover the integrity of the skin's outer layer, which is called the stratum corneum
- Recover the integrity of the precious hydrolipid barrier that enables the skin to retain water, fight wrinkles, and keep out harmful chemicals

- Recover uninterrupted function of the skin's bacteria-fighting surface acidity, known as its acid mantle

Once we get back these basic components of "virgin skin," we can have a far greater success rate in identifying the real solutions for our skin—if we still need them. For some, merely stopping the assaults to basic skin function is all it takes for their skin to fully recover.

The Stratum Corneum: The Gatekeeper of Beautiful Skin

The skin's outer layer is called the stratum corneum. Since the emergence of alpha-hydroxy acids in the mid-1990s, the trend in skin care has been to penetrate and break this layer to reveal plump, healthy skin. But this outer layer contains most of the skin's anti-aging, antiwrinkling, and anti-bacterial protection, and it is the skin's primary sunscreen. Immature cells beneath the surface need the protection of this outer layer to develop properly and be healthy when they arrive at the surface. Recovering and maintaining the stratum corneum will optimize your skin's pro-beauty function and ecology. It is a necessary first step if you want a shot at perfect, low-maintenence skin.

The Hydrolipid Barrier

The skin depends on the hydrolipid barrier to retain water. It is the skin's waterproof seal that was never meant to be broken but is commonly destroyed by modern, high-tech skin-care regimens. The barrier is a primary defense against foreign substances, drying, and wrinkling.

The Acid Mantle

The skin's acid mantle, made of sweat, mature skin cells, bacteria, and sebum, is the optimum surface skin environment. It sounds like something we should get rid of altogether, but the acid mantle is the naturally low pH skin surface that protects the skin against infectious bacteria—and thus acne and other irritations. It can easily be obliterated by skin products that contain detergents, soaps, or antiseptics, and in many women—and even teens!—it is never given a chance to recover or perform its intended function. Its absence inevitably leads to skin problems that can only be controlled but never resolved until we restore the acid mantle.

what disrupts normal skin-cell function

Alpha-Hydroxy Acids

Alpha-hydroxy acids (AHAs)—the popular skin-exfoliating acids including glycolic, citric, malic, and lactic acids—are prevalent in mainstream cleansers, moisturizers, toners, and even makeup. Several prominent skin experts over the years have expressed concerns that continued use of AHAs could compromise the skin's protective functions. The FDA is currently investigating concerns that AHAs—which have never been studied long-term—might damage DNA by increasing sun exposure and promote skin cancer. In an interview with *Fashion Wire Daily*, Dr. Lynn Drake, chief of dermatology at the University of Oklahoma and past president of the American Academy of Dermatology, said, "We honestly don't know the long-term effects of alpha hydroxy acids on the skin. The body has a mechanism for rejuvenating the skin automatically. With AHAs, I'm concerned that we are going to change the normal biorhythms of the skin."

Over-exfoliating

Over-exfoliating with AHAs as well as other physical exfoliants, such as cleansing grains and scrubs, ages and sensitizes the skin by

- Abrading, tearing, and sensitizing the skin
- Dramatically increasing the skin's vulnerability to sun damage
- Destroying the hydrolipid barrier

- Compromising the acid mantle
- Making it vulnerable to chemicals it was never intended to absorb

And while keeping acne-prone skin clear of debris is important, any irritating exfoliating product can aggravate inflammation. If full-blown acne is the issue, then working your way down to the mildest exfoliation products and removing as many irritating ingredients from them as possible will help you recover your skin's natural defenses.

To wean yourself off of AHAs and other exfoliants, use antimicrobial essential oils for acne as well as gentle but effective antioxidant and marine-extract serums to stimulate cell renewal and collagen production for wrinkle reversal and prevention. See chapter 11 and the Resources for further recommendations.

Oil-Stripping and Drying Regimens

Virtually all soaps, foaming cleansers, and alcohol-based toners, with the exception of cetyl and cetearyl alcohols, which are not drying like other alcohols, will compromise the skin's hydrolipid barrier. Many of these cleansers contain solvents, such as sodium lauryl sulfate, that can cause the skin to lose water and protein and become rough, sensitive, and prone to premature wrinkling, particularly when included in skin and shampoo formulas at concentrations greater then 1 percent—and the only way to find this out is to ask the manufacturer. These products often leave the skin feeling tight—which is a sign that it's been stripped—and often cause it to produce more oil in a rebound effort to regulate its own moisture. But even after the sebum returns, the skin's barrier and bacterial balance remain compromised, and blemishes and other inflammatory problems are more likely to occur until the barrier is reestablished. This will require the discontinuation of soap and solvent-based degreasing cleansers. On a purely aesthetic note, when the skin surface is dried up and deprived of its own lubrication, blemishes often stop moving through the skin and remain suspended beneath the surface for prolonged periods. Peeling often alternates with or accompanies oiliness. Blemishes spot-zapped with benzoyl peroxide

ANTIBACTERIAL SOAPS AND ANTIBIOTIC SKIN TREATMENTS

Most dermatologists regard antibacterial soaps as not only overkill but also potentially dangerous since they destroy beneficial bacteria and can create resistant bacteria—even in people who live with those who use them. Whether you're using over-the-counter antibacterial soaps or an antibiotic regimen from your dermatologist, you run a risk of developing resistant bacteria and the certainty that you will be more vulnerable to breakouts and other negative skin effects caused by pathogenic bacteria between uses. Oral antibiotics dramatically increase these risks throughout the body and can lead to dandruff, yeast infections, toe and nail fungus, and itchy, uncomfortable skin. They can also impair digestion and absorption of nutrients and give rise to possible lifelong sensitivities, allergies, and auto-immune issues that affect the skin and the entire body. If you're taking prescription antibiotics for a chronic skin problem, discuss with your doctor topically applied options as an interim upgrade and the possibility of weaning off of them completely. During the weaning process you can minimize a recurrence of infectious skin problems by incorporating natural antimicrobial topicals (discussed in chapter 11), which have not been shown to create resistant bacteria, into your skin-care regimen. Also use the skin-supportive feeding and cultivating suggestions in part II, which can influence your resistance to harmful bacteria not only in the skin but also throughout the entire body.

become crusty, unattractive, and harder to cover. Foundation appears blotchy and unnatural. Don't destroy the beauty of your skin for the sake of temporary clarity!

spare your skin by upgrading your morning shower

What if you could dramatically improve the health and beauty of your skin and hair, reduce your allergies and your risk of cancer, and eliminate a daily source of premature aging and needless toxic exposure without altering your routine? It's as simple as installing a filter on your showerhead.

Most people are unaware of the countless ways that chlorinated shower water can undermine their efforts at beautiful skin, hair, and health. By compromising the skin's bacteria-fighting acid mantle and protective barrier and then penetrating and causing oxidative damage, chlorine represents a huge cumulative skin burden, making normal to dry skin sensitive, dryer, and more vulnerable to irritation, dandruff, and fungal infections. And if the skin is already stripped, dry, or rough, your daily shower can devastate it. Chlorine also contributes to dry, brittle hair and scalp. And if you color your hair, there's the nuisance of chlorine's mild bleaching effect.

But there are even more important reasons to make this painless and inexpensive adjustment. Our pores soak chlorine directly into the bloodstream. According to research conducted jointly at Harvard University and the Medical College of Wisconsin, chlorinated water contributes to 9 percent of all bladder cancers and 18 percent of all rectal cancers in the United States.

Furthermore, the heat in your shower produces chloroform from the water, which—when inhaled—can aggravate allergies, respiratory and sinus conditions, and asthma. These issues can cause under-eye puffiness and circles.

The humble shower filter might just be the biggest beauty and health bang for the buck there is. To set yourself up with affordable yet quality filtration, look for the newer zinc-copper filter technology, which works with heat much better than the old carbon filters (see the Resources).

stop stripping the skin and start purifying it

The most renowned beauty oils—among them jojoba, apricot kernel, sweet almond, squalene, and emu—are noted for their similarity to sebum, nature's perfect lubricant. The best shampoos are considered such because they "replenish" natural sheen to the hair, *which they've just stripped*. Many find it hard to grasp that it is not necessary to dissolve every trace of sebum in order to "start fresh." There are a number of effective ways to cleanse and purify the skin without stripping it. Various cleansers containing natural antimicrobial essential oils and substances can deeply purify the sebum and even help normalize its production without compromising the skin's hydrolipid barrier or causing breakouts. See chapter 11 and the Resources for some of the substances and products I recommend.

THE BABY-WIPE TRICK, ONLY BETTER

Whenever I do makeup for the New York fashion shows, I use baby wipes. It's a popular trick to quickly clean makeup off of models' faces. They work well, but the perfumes and other potential irritants in your average baby wipe aren't something you'd want on your face very often. Fortunately, not all baby wipes are created equal. Baby wipes available at health-food stores are aloe-based and free of fragrance and propylene glycol. They are a far healthier way to wash your face than most forty-dollar fancy cleansers you could buy at the department store.

tone down your toner

If you're using a cleanser that contains a lot of petrochemicals (fragrance, colors, propylene glycol, mineral oil), which sit on or irritate the skin, it makes sense to take an extra step to make sure the residue is removed, but not if that means using a toner filled with nasty pollutants and irritants. And if you're cleansing with substances that actually purify and nourish the skin, there is little need for a toner at all. In the morning, however, when your face is essentially clean, you may want to use toner to remove any oil or dirt it has accumulated overnight before you apply light moisturizers or serums and then makeup. Even if your skin is quite oily, fight the urge to strip it in the morning with foaming cleansers and alcohol-based, drying toners. Go for a purifying ritual that leaves the skin's oils intact.

You can easily make a toner that keeps in the fridge for a week. Use aloe juice (healing and anti-inflammatory); a dash of apple-cider vinegar (restores optimum pH); a generous splash of strong green, chamomile, or licorice tea (anti-inflammatory and antioxidant); and a few drops of lavender essential oil (antimicrobial and calming). Add a few drops of tea tree oil, neem oil, or grapefruit-seed extract for stronger antibacterial action. If you don't have time for home recipes, check out the alcohol-free toners at the

MY MORNING TEA-BAG TRICK

After I make my daily pot of green (or licorice or chamomile) tea using purified water, I save the tea bags in a closed glass container in the fridge and use them as little cleansing pads the next morning. They're perfect for a little exfoliation. Tea has anti-inflammatory properties and zero negatives to challenge your skin. If you have acne-prone skin that may require slightly deeper cleaning, use a washcloth moistened with tea and a dot of the right cleanser or essential oil (see chapter 11).

Save deeper cleansing for evenings, when there's makeup to remove. Mornings don't have to be scary for your skin!

health-food store. When choosing a toner, avoid potentially drying or disruptive ingredients, like fragrance, propylene glycol, sulfates, and alcohols (other than ceteryl or cetyl).

the only way to rebuild the skin's barrier

Letting the skin barrier recover once it's been stripped can take days to a couple of weeks, depending on the degree of damage, but we can speed the process with carefully selected topical tactics. Phospholipids derived primarily from soy and egg yolks are the only substances that possess the ability to directly rebuild the hydrolipid barrier when applied topically. They protect your skin and become a part of the skin-cell membranes. They are able to form liposomes, which can nourish the skin and deliver EFAs, such as linoleic acid. Linoleic acid can rebuild the lipid barrier to prevent water loss and dry skin. At the same time it can reduce overproduction of oil and inhibit acne. See the Resources for products containing phospholipids and EFAs.

DON'T DEPRIVE YOUR SKIN WITH DENATURED OILS

Just as stripped foods seriously deprive the body, stripped and refined oils may seriously deprive your skin. EFAs are found in cold-pressed, skin-compatible oils, but they are lost once those oils are refined or tampered with. Mineral oil and petrolatum are highly refined petrochemical derivatives that, according to phytochemist Aubrey Hampton, Ph.D., can actually leave the skin and the lips dryer because they block sebum's crucial functions and interfere with the skin's ability to regulate its own moisture. And both mineral oil and petrolatum have been shown to cause chemically induced acne.

the recovery and restraint period: resist the "do something" impulse

Once you've discontinued your harsh products and incorporated the inside-out regimen upgrades in this book, you should see a marked decrease in skin sensitivity in anywhere from a few weeks to only a few days, depending on the harshness of your original regimen. You will also see an increase in skin activity, as blemishes suspended beneath the skin may move to surface and live out their destiny over the next couple of weeks. As the skin surface recovers its integrity, makeup will go on more smoothly and last longer. Sensitivity and ruddiness will subside. Skin problems may seem worse for a few days or even a couple weeks before they get better, but you can minimize this rebound period by immediately incorporating skin-supportive product, beverage, food, supplement, and even emotional regimens. The sum of this holistic approach will change your skin in ways your old harsh regimens never could.

treat your hair like your skin

Our hair may be not be alive, but that doesn't keep us from killing it. Like fine leather, how we wash and care for our hair makes a world of difference in its quality and luster. Because hair can only be cosmetically altered once it has been harmed—although, luckily, damage grows out—it's important to cultivate resilient, strong hair via healthier scalp and hair follicles by feeding them from within and avoiding the very same stripping, irritating, and drying assaults that cause problems on the skin.

Tricks and Tweaks That Spare Your Hair

Don't over-wash your hair. If you have oily hair and wash it every day, don't wash twice, and don't lather the ends. If you have dry hair, don't wash more than twice a week, unless you use one of the non-foaming radical hair-cleansing techniques (see sidebar) or gentler shampoo options such as those listed in the Resources. If your scalp is itchy, wash more often, but keep in mind that dandruff and itching may clear up once you install a shower filter, change your products, optimize your body's probiotic ecology, and start eating better food. You know you've achieved healthy internal ecology when your scalp stops itching, even when it's oily.

RADICAL SHAMPOO-LESS HAIR-CLEANSING TECHNIQUES

Can hair truly be cleaned without foaming cleansers or shampoo? It absolutely can. In fact, your hair can be softer and your scalp healthier than you ever imagined if you stop using or minimize your use of shampoo. The list of celebrity enthusiasts for L.A. hair pro Chaz Dean's Wen line of hair products is almost as impressive as his famous cleansing conditioner. The tea tree formula purifies the scalp and hair with essential oils. Another non-foaming product that uses essential oils as well as clay-based minerals is Terressentials Hair Wash. You can use these products exclusively or alternate with sulfate-free, ultra-gentle shampoos such as those listed in the Resources.

Dry Your Hair Smartly

Dry your hair naturally (see the bodifying technique following) or use a super-absorbent hair chamois. Infrared or ionic blow-dryers also minimize damage by drying hair evenly, inside and out, rather than scorching the outer cuticle layer, which is frayed by conventional dryers (see the Resources).

How to Get Body without Stressing Your Hair

Wash or wet your hair in the evening. After gently squeezing (never rubbing) wet hair with a super-absorbent hair chamois, apply a touch of leave-in conditioner or moisturizer by first raking through your hair with your hands, concentrating on the ends, and then using a wide-tooth comb to distribute. If your hair is wavy, let it dry naturally. If your hair is straight and long enough, bend over and gently comb your hair straight up, working the comb from ends to roots so as not to force it through any tangles, then twist your hair to make a loose bun on top of your head and secure with a cotton scrunchie. Sleep with your hair this way. When you let it down in the morning, you will have the body and wave you've always dreamed of. For more wave, try spraying NaPCA into your hair after using the chamois; it draws moisture into the hair without weighing it down.

WHAT'S GOOD FOR THE SKIN IS GOOD FOR THE HAIR

When applied sparingly, the moisturizers that are most ideal for your type of hair are often the same moisturizers and oils that work best on your skin. Some of the more expensive ingredients serve no purpose in your hair, but the basic natural moisturizers make great texturizing products. Moisturizers that penetrate the skin without leaving a greasy film are great for both oily skin and the hair type that generally comes with it. Dry hair responds wonderfully to the same textured creams for dry skin. Distribute a dab of moisturizer on your hands by rubbing them together and apply it to hair ends only at first.

Avoid a Harsh Cut

A cut should yield to your features and softly frame them, not compete with them. Cutting with a razor or a slithered or texturized scissor can create wave, lift, and movement and give you lower-maintenance hair. Let your hair change from day to day. Let it have its own life. Refrain from conquering your hair and showing it who's boss. Letting your hair do its own thing will lead you to the best cut. It can also improve your self-image.

give yourself a permanent break from harsh self-treatment

We need to stop being harsh on ourselves. Stop using soaps that dry, blemish creams that irritate, lotions that sting, shampoos that strip, chemical-laden perfumes that poison, and exfoliants that leave your skin raw. As you begin to support your skin from within, you can begin to sit back and let your body deal with and heal each passing skin issue and see how a little restraint and the world of inside-out strategies can turn irritated skin into calm, glowing skin and chronic issues into transient ones that no longer cause panic.

Chapter 10

PURIFY YOUR POTIONS AND PAINTS

We don't need to aspire to know everything about cosmetic ingredients to set an informed criterion for what we use on our bodies, but in order to shed the true irritants and toxins that can burden your skin and your health, it is imperative to get a basic understanding of what you put on your body day in and day out. Some of it affects your skin's beauty, and some of it could be affecting your vitality and your hormonal state as well as your future.

Perhaps the most realistic approach is for you to fully understand the degree of your current vulnerability. The amount of crucial information that goes unreported and undetected on labels due to the lack of testing requirements and effective regulation is astounding. Holes in your understanding could be setting you up for skin and health problems that are hard to trace. Let's close up some of those holes.

what goes on, goes in

Back in beauty school, "product safety" meant not getting perm solution in your client's eyes. We learned how to pronounce and spell chemical names. We learned how they could change hair structure. We learned how to protect our hands with gloves. But we never learned about the possible proven effects of long-term exposure to some of the concoctions we slathered on our clients. At enrollment they don't tell you that cosmetologists develop multiple myeloma—a form of bone-marrow cancer—at four times the rate of the general population. This fact is more widely known to health insurers than to a budding beautician or the women she applies these chemical onto.

Skin absorption is now widely recognized as a significant way for substances to enter the body. In some cases it provides even more passage into the bloodstream than eating or drinking. Some scientists estimate that as much as 60 percent of what we apply on our skin winds up in our bloodstream.

There is a growing concern about the accumulation of estrogen-mimicking chemicals in the breast tissues of women and in the prostate tissues of men. Just about every day, a new industrial or cosmetic chemical or chemical combination is found to be a hormone-disrupting substance. Hormone disruption can cause uterine cell changes, cell proliferation, and other signs of elevated estrogen activity. Estrogen dominance is becoming more prevalent in this country and contributes to breast cancer and reproductive and weight problems. Hormone imposters are a compelling place to start with regard to cosmetic ingredients.

Phthalates, a type of chemical used in nail polish and hair spray, are confirmed estrogen mimics of growing concern to the Centers for Disease Control (CDC). The CDC has discovered forty-five times more phthalates (particularly dibutyl phthalate, found in nail polish) in women ages twenty to forty than previously estimated. A recent study found that many of the most commonly used synthetic sunscreen ingredients, including benzophenone-3 and octyl-methoxy-cinnamates (OMC), accumulate in the breast milk and organs of rats, producing estrogenic effects, which researchers say suggests it may have the same effects in humans. The common preservatives methyl, propyl, butyl and ethyl paraben, long thought to be safe synthetic preservatives, were found to be mildly estrogenic in a 1998 study in which researchers concluded that "given their use in a wide range of commercially available topical preparations, it is suggested that the safety in use of these chemicals should be reassessed."

The medical industry has jumped on the concept of transdermal patches that deliver drugs directly into the bloodstream, but the cosmetics industry chooses whether to emphasize if a product is absorbed by the skin. In the case of vitamin C crows-feet patches, skin absorption is stressed, but when it comes to coal-tar dyes in color cosmetics and in hair color, for example, you are unlikely to hear the claim "penetrates deep," even though they do.

the threshold principle

Each of us has a threshold at which we react not just to any one irritant but also to the number of irritants we are exposed to at a given time. And any additional exposure we encounter once we reach our saturation point could make us suddenly quite sensitive and even chronically sick. For example, formaldehyde, which can be found in all sorts of cosmetics—as well as in food, new clothes, and fumes in our homes—can build up in the body without causing acute symptoms before suddenly reaching a saturation point at which a person becomes sensitive to even minute amounts, according to Angel DeFazio, B.Sci., A.T., president of the National Toxic Encephalopathy Foundation.

The threshold principle also applies to allergic responses. Exposure to sensitizing substances over a long period of time or too many allergens at once can cause a reaction to a substance you may never have reacted to in the past.

Remember, though, that just because a substance is natural doesn't mean it won't cause a reaction in some people. Essential oils with therapeutic effects on one person can cause an allergic reaction in another (which is why a patch test is a good idea before incorporating them into your regimens). Studies have linked talc with asbestos contamination and cancer. The popular diet herb ephedra can cause heart problems. But unlike synthetically derived chemicals, few, if any, naturally occurring substances have been found to accumulate in the body and in the environment indefinitely. Natural antimicrobials, which are often similar and, in some cases, superior in power to antibiotics, have not been shown to produce resistant strains of bacteria as synthetics can. Many scientists believe this is because natural antimicrobials are much more complex than synthetics in their mechanisms of action and therefore cannot be adapted to by bacteria.

how regulation doesn't work

In a 1994 study published in the *Journal of the National Cancer Institute*, researchers examined the relationship between the use of permanent hair dyes and selected fatal cancers in 573,369 women and concluded that women who use black hair dyes over a long period of time may have an increased risk of fatal non-Hodgkin's lymphoma and multiple myeloma. Researchers urged that "the removal of carcinogens from hair dyes and appropriate labeling of hair-coloring products would help reduce this potential risk." But a prior attempt by the FDA to require a warning label on permanent hair-coloring products after studies showed certain ingredients to be mutagenic in the late 1970s was thwarted by a regulatory loophole that exempted these ingredients from the FDA's jurisdiction. These products remain on the shelf today, in spite of recent studies indicating that they may cause bladder cancer in humans. Many other countries, including Japan, have banned carcinogenic hair-color ingredients, the most notorious of which is phenylenediamine (PPD).

Some coal tar colors (F,D,&C or D&C dyes used in hair color, makeup, and skin-care products) that have been tested were shown to cause cancer when injected into the skin of rodents, and yet most have never been adequately tested for safety in cosmetic use. We do know they can cause acne and allergies, but whatever else they cause is anyone's guess. This is true of most cosmetics ingredients. In fact, experts from the National Research Council and the National Academy of Science who were involved with one of the first large government studies of cosmetic ingredients in 1984 concluded that "of the tens of thousands of commercially important chemicals, only a few have been subjected to extensive toxicity testing and most have scarcely been tested at all."

While the government does actually require a warning label on products that have not been adequately tested, there is no congressional mandate for this, so the industry has not complied. The FDA spends less than 1 percent of its budget on supervising the industry. The Cosmetic, Toiletry, and Fragrance Association (CTFA) acts as both the effective regulator as well as the special interest and key lobbying organization on the industry's behalf. The Cosmetic Ingredient Review (CIR), a small group of experts that reviews thousands of cosmetics ingredients, is largely funded by the CTFA, and relies mostly on unpublished data, according to Judi Vance, publisher of *Cosmetic Health Report* and author of *Beauty to Die For*. This is just a small sample of the loopholes, delays, appeals, inactions, conflicts of interest, and exemptions that riddle cosmetic regulation and render it all but useless or worse, since it provides a false sense of security. If you want more insight into the circus of cosmetic regulation, see the Resources for suggested reading.

if it's not the chemical itself, it's the contaminants, by-products, and combinations

One of the major inherent problems with synthesized cosmetic materials is that they tend to be contaminated or to form by-products during manufacturing or storage or while on the skin. For example, the cosmetic chemicals listed on labels as TEA, DEA, and MEA or their full names, which end in "amine," like triethanolamine, were found in 1998 by the National Toxicology Program (NTP) to form nitrosamines, which cause cancer in mice. PEG, or polyethylene glycol, a common synthetic emollient, is often contaminated with dioxane, another known hormone disruptor and a carcinogen that the Consumer Product Safety Commission has determined to be dangerous even at low-level exposure. Quaternium-15, a common cosmetic preservative, can release formaldehyde, another carcinogen, and cause skin reactions. Formaldehyde, widely known to be one of the most dangerous common chemicals, is used in nail polish and in all kinds of synthetic hair-, skin-, and body-care products as an antimicrobial and preservative, but it is never listed on the label as "formaldehyde." It has dozens of aliases (most have the word "form" in it, like "formalin," "lysoform," and "formalith"), but they're not always listed, since other chemicals can release formaldehyde as a by-product, such as imidazolidinyl urea, a common preservative in shampoos, when they reach certain temperatures.

If the formaldehyde and dibutyl phthalate don't make nail polish scary enough, there's the other key ingredient, toluene, which can cause rashes, neurological symptoms, and harm to the kidneys and liver during frequent use, according to both the EPA and the U.S. Department of Health and Human Services Agency for Toxic Substances and Disease Registry. Thankfully, professional-grade polish without the three most infamous ingredients is now available.

perfume or pollutant: another major unknown

I once sat on an airplane next to a woman who got up and then returned from the restroom reeking of perfume. She sat there sniffling and messing up her perfect makeup with the tissue she used to repeatedly dab her nose and eyes. It was like looking at myself when I was twenty. Many people are sensitive to the very fragrances they use on themselves every day. In fact, fragrance is one of the top contact allergens and often contains petroleum-based chemicals identified as carcinogens and neurotoxins, according to the National Academy of Sciences.

Analysis has shown that some seriously harmful ingredients are showing up in even the finest perfumes. According to Samuel Epstein, M.D., Professor of Environmental Medicine at the University of Illinois School of Public Health, Chicago, a recent analysis of one of the most famous designer perfumes revealed forty-one ingredients, including some known to be toxic to the skin, respiratory tract, and nervous and reproductive systems. Data about toxicity were either unavailable or inadequate on several of the ingredients. Additionally, some ingredients were determined to be volatile and sources of indoor air pollution.

Allergies to fragrance grew more prevalent in the United States from the 1980s to 1990s. In conventional skin and hair products, fragrance is impossible to avoid, since it is allowed even in products labeled "fragrance free." Therefore, we can only knowingly escape from fragrance by using products with essential oil–based scents or products that are 100 percent certified organic.

what's in a label

Most of us know not to trust labels on a conscious level, and yet many of us tend to suspend our disbelief if the packaging, smell, and marketing strike our fancy. But even the term "made with 100 percent pure extracts" can appear on the poetic packaging of what is really a plastic, synthetic concoction. "Natural" may not actually mean natural. Furthermore, "hypoallergenic" does not mean you won't react to a product; it is a phrase for which manufacturers have their own interpretations. Here's another caveat: Hypoallergenic products are allowed to contain fragrance even if the label states "fragrance-free." And "non-comedogenic" is yet another unregulated term that tells you nothing. Mineral oil, which has been shown to cause chemically induced acne, appears in some supposedly non-comedogenic products. "Dermatologist tested" can mean anything and nothing. Any dermatologist with any motive or vested interest can test a product, but the results of the test don't have to be scientific or even positive. There are no regulations setting any standard meaning for any of these terms. The term "pH-balanced" can actually indicate harmful products, according to Dr. Aubrey Hampton, who says that triethanolamine (TEA), the substance that forms cancer-causing nitrosamines, is often used in cosmetics to adjust their pH levels.

Personally, I don't spend a lot of time deciphering hard-to-pronounce ingredient lists anymore because I rarely deal with products that bear them. Even if there weren't inherent risks in synthetic chemical combinations and the serious lack of testing, I would not want to deny myself the therapeutic actions, purity, and life force of naturally occurring, biologically active substances. Those who are ill or chemically sensitive may choose to avoid the risks of synthesized chemicals altogether, and those who are concerned about the environment will surely take all this into account in setting their own criterion for what goes on—and in—their bodies and down their drains. Getting informed allows you to choose your potions consistently with your values.

"organic" on labels: deciphering the lingering loopholes

The USDA's National Organic Rule (NOR) on organic standards for foods went into effect in October 2002 and was a landmark regulation that gave full credibility to the word *organic* on food labels. It assures consumers that foods labeled "100 percent organic" are completely free of pesticides, hormones, antibiotics, chemical fertilizers, irradiation, and genetically modified ingredients.

But the USDA does not regulate personal-care products and there are no standards set in stone. Most health-food stores won't sell products with synthetic perfumes, colors, or mineral oil, and while it is possible to learn which ingredients are organic by reading the ingredients list, some companies count the high percentage of "organic" floral water they use (listed as "hydrosols") toward the total organic content of the product, and you could wind up using products that still contain a lot of synthetics in the remaining percentage of ingredients. The industry is working on establishing standards as I write this, but for now, one cannot trust the term *organic* on the front label of hair and skincare products—only on the ingredients list, if the listing is certified. Some natural products that aren't organic may be purer than some organic ones.

The German certification for natural products, BIDH, is quite similar to the USDA's NOR, with a few additional ethical recommendations, such as no animal testing and emphasis on using ingredients from fair-trade and third-world projects. European products often use the word "fragrance" on their labels, even if natural plant essences are used.

don't be seduced by the pseudonaturals

Because of our desire to reconnect with nature, we are prone to accept pseudonatural products. From products that include token natural botanicals and fake aromatherapy candles that are actually toxic to inhale, to flowery yet synthetic body lotions made by "green-conscious" companies, to the most luxuriously packaged and ingeniously marketed "real imposters" that smell of lavender or green tea—there is no such thing as essence of green tea, by the way—we are entering a new phase of sensory exploitation. The ingredients are no different from those used in the fruity concoctions of the 1980s, but the marketing is much more brilliant. Its success in exploiting both our senses and our sensibilities relies on one key condition: that we as individuals remain uninformed and don't look at the ingredients list.

It is exciting to remove that shiny box from that chichi little shopping bag, but your body doesn't care about the packaging. Once you've tossed the fancy foil box, the cellophane, and the rest of the cardboard, you're probably still getting plastic inside the bottle. Why apply a dead and perfumed product in a beautiful package when you can use one that can give you its life force in perfect harmony with your body and the environment?

There are a lot of intelligent, self-respecting women who'd be shocked to know the degree to which they've been duped into accepting cheaply made, irritating concoctions as the cutting edge in skin care. All too often a few beneficial or even patented breakthrough ingredients are carried in a soup of known irritants included primarily to benefit the manufacturer. Drug- and department-store brands generally contain only 5 to 8 percent active ingredients, yet ads can go on and on about the effectiveness of those ingredients. And even if they do use the amount proven to have a clinical effect, the rest of what's in the bottle may be a synthetic gravy.

The longer we immerse ourselves in fake tastes and smells, the more we lose our ability to decipher what's real. But even if you can't tell the difference between an essential oil of lavender and lavender-scented solvents and petrochemicals, your *body* knows. Just as it is offended by the denatured matter we are presented with as food, our bodies are offended by these chemicals posing as true substance.

Nature's prohibitive cost to manufacturers due to the care required in extracting, storing, and delivering its inimitable rewards has united mainstream manufacturers in an unspoken pact not to let on that truly natural products are possible to produce. The more dirt-cheap synthetics you use and the harsher and more prevalent the preservatives, the longer your product will last, the cheaper it is to make, and the higher the profit, and thus the more the manufacturer can spend on packaging, the more beautiful and prominent their ads can be, and the more exciting—yet worthless—that beautifully packaged product will be to the consumer.

enter microbrewed cosmetics: substance over packaging

A growing number of skin companies are doing what the synthetic skin-care giants claimed was impossible. These microchemists are saying no to mass production and warehousing protocol and are giving up vast profits to create biologically active skin- and body-care products that contain live, unadulterated ingredients. Like microbrewed beer, cosmetic products produced in small batches are likely to contain few, if any, harmful ingredients. These companies often use essential oils and citrus-seed extract as preservatives, and if they use any synthetics, they are in the most minute amounts. These products are significantly more expensive to produce, and the value of the natural substances used is hard to quantify. Without patent profits behind them, you're unlikely to see these products advertised in your favorite magazines or on television, but among their cult followers, including celebrities and fashionistas, microbrewed cosmetics are fast gaining appeal and the long-awaited acknowledgment they truly deserve. Fresh-product boutiques, beauty bars, Internet companies with no warehousing that send out fresh products as you order them, and mom-and-pop companies that mix up fresh concoctions are becoming the rage. You can find these products at your local natural-food stores. Look for them in specialty stores, read more about them in editorials in your favorite magazines, and of course, surf the Internet.

my criterion

Choosing products is easy for me because I set my pure, potent, and proven criterion long ago. I'm not a purist by any means, and I will use commercial products on occasion for a temporary effect. People always ask me about specific brand names. I don't enchant myself with brands or fancy marketing because they're meaningless. Look at the ingredients list; that's what counts. Some companies have amazing integrity, but all of their products might not be right for you. Don't be afraid to use a serum from one company and a cleanser from another or to alternate and evolve your products with your skin's fluctuations. It's about you, not brand loyalty. Now that you have the facts, you can set your own standards and find products that deliver the purity and potency you crave.

Purity is the new decadence.

Finally, whether you're dealing with food or with beauty and body products, always demand full disclosure. It's the very least you can do for yourself, since any product you use will become a part of you.

Chapter 11

STRATEGIZE A WHOLE NEW SKIN APPROACH

An inside-out approach to preventing and dealing with possible causes for skin distress will have far more impact than external care alone. Broadening your understanding of the possible issues that connect your lifestyle with your skin can save you a lifetime of wasted energy and dollars on futile treatments and save your skin the perpetual ravages of regimen overkill. The work associated with high-maintenance skin regimens seems necessary but may be in vain if the true cause of the problem is not being addressed. Getting to the cause doesn't take work; it takes information, self-knowledge, and a passion for becoming your own connoisseur. When you have truly established a cause and strategized against the cause alone (while restraining from problem-causing quick fixes), you'll be on your way to a true resolution. Best of all, addressing that cause and correcting that imbalance will make the rest of you more radiant, too.

For example, if you discover that your thyroid isn't working properly, you open a door to possibly curing your dry skin—and your weight issue. If you suffer from dandruff and itchy skin and bring back the pro-beauty, good-bacteria ecology in your gut, you might save yourself a lifetime of black-sweater avoidance, dandruff shampoos, skin eruptions, and a future of more serious compounded health problems.

GETTING MORE THAN A PRESCRIPTION OUT OF YOUR TRIP TO THE DERMATOLOGIST

Symptom-focused quick fixes may get us out of the doctor's office in ten minutes, but they often keep us going back. Here is how you can get the most out of your trip to the dermatologist:

- Consider going in for diagnosis only unless you need to get something removed or biopsied. Tell your dermatologist up front that your goal is to understand what's wrong, not to walk out with a prescription.
- Take your medical records with you so you have a better chance of getting to the cause of your skin condition.
- Take with you your list of symptoms beyond what your doctor will be able to see from your skin. Include the products and/or conditions that seem to exacerbate the problem.
- List any prescription drugs you're taking and discuss possible skin-related side effects.
- Involve your primary-care physician or a nutrition-oriented physician if a skin condition is chronic.

A dermatologist can help you properly diagnose your skin condition, but you may need to do some work on your own or with your doctor to identify the day-to-day personal habits, treatments, and triggers behind your skin issues. Always factor in what you're putting on or into your body, any medications you are taking, and your emotional state. The dawn-to-dusk self-inventory you took earlier in the book can help you identify patterns and choices that may contribute to your skin issues. Regular health exams can help rule out or pinpoint any health issues that affect your skin, like hormonal imbalances, auto-immune syndromes, systemic yeast, nutritional imbalances, hydration, sleep disturbances, environmental sensitivities, liver and thyroid function, stress, and prescription-drug side effects.

Many chronic skin conditions can be improved and even reversed if these causes are addressed at the start rather than as a last resort, lest you pile on harsher regimens or drugs and complicate matters in an attempt to overcome issues that just can't be fixed at the surface. It's much harder to pinpoint the cause or even diagnose the real problem once it is compounded with treatments that compromise the skin's function and cause new imbalances.

The closer you are to achieving nutritional, hormonal, emotional, and digestive balance, the closer you are to healthy skin. Remember that all healthy skin is vulnerable to wild cards, like food additives, contact irritants, and prescription medications. If these issues are affecting your skin now, years of practicing the latest treatments and surface approaches won't help.

the brief history and exciting future of truly effective skin care

The detailed chart found at the end of this chapter will open up a world of greater vitality and radiance to be gained by looking at the big picture of your skin issues as they relate to possible health and lifestyle factors. But before that, let's look at some new stars on the beauty scene that represent the future of skin care. These products and remedies are hot, not because they are new substances but because they are backed by new proof for what is, in many cases, ancient knowledge being relearned and technically applied by an intuition-challenged modern society.

Until the early 1990s, there was little offered by skin-care technology but temporary surface-texture enhancement and protection from sun and dehydration. Vitamins and botanicals were used primarily as a marketing concept but not taken seriously by any self-respecting dermatologist. And consumers had grown desensitized to the glowing promises in skin-care ads. But then came Retin A, alpha-hydroxy acids, and the first science showing that vitamin C could stimulate collagen production when applied topically. From that point on, skin care—and the attitude toward natural substances—would never be the same. Now it seems that each passing day brings more scientific evidence of what can be done to reverse past damage and change the current function of our skin simply by taking or applying a natural substance. The ongoing challenge has been in effectively stabilizing and delivering these substances to the skin before they lose their effect. And if the steady stream of science proving the efficacy of more and more topically applied antioxidants and botanicals is any indication, those challenges are being successfully met. Here are the main categories of effective skin-care ingredients and the science-backed stars of each.

Potent Antioxidants and Anti-inflammatories

Zinc, green tea, milk thistle, curcumin, vitamin C, tocotrienols, alpha-lipoic acid, superoxide dismutase (S.O.D.), CoQ10, and pycnogenol have all demonstrated both antioxidant and anti-inflammatory action in scientific studies. They scavenge the free radicals that lead to wrinkles and precancerous cell changes. Vitamin C has shown perhaps the most compelling proof as a collagen-building wrinkle-reverser. Green, black, and white teas have been found to inhibit inflammation and sun damage. Licorice and chamomile have demonstrated long-term anti-inflammatory action similar to topical steroids without the side-effects. Even good old aloe is now proven to be a powerful anti-inflammatory and healer with mild collagen-building and antiseptic properties. It contains salicylic acid, which explains the pain-killing effects when applied to sunburns.

Beyond antioxidants, there's a promising new crop of wrinkle-reversers in this post–alpha-hydroxy acid beauty world, including Kinetin or Kinerase products, featuring the growth factor furfuryladenine (which can diminish wrinkles without irritation), the anti-glycation substance carnosine, and even a drinkable form of collagen. Marine extracts are the other class of substances that holds the most promise to rejuvenate the skin.

See the Resources for products containing these ingredients. They are just the tip of the iceberg of what is to emerge in the growing body of science-validated natural substances over the next few years.

Plant Phospholipids

Phospholipids are important components of the skin's natural protective barrier. Detergents and solvents in skin products can compromise this natural protection in the skin, but topically applied plant phospholipids have been shown to restore the skin's own membrane and literally become part of the skin after exposure to detergents and solvents. Phospholipids also act as a humectant, while preventing water evaporation. They are the only substance that can form liposomes, arguably the most important breakthrough in skin treatment today. Liposomes can carry nourishment into the skin cells and even create reservoirs of moisture deep within the skin, which is not possible with other treatments.

Cold-Pressed Oils and EFAs

I had extremely dry skin until my late twenties. EFAs like flax, evening primrose, borage, and fish oil normalized my skin. When I first took EFA supplements for my liver, I didn't understand their multitude of serious beauty benefits. For example, gamma-linolenic acid (GLA), a type of EFA from evening-primrose and borage oils, inhibits an androgen-related enzyme that promotes oily skin, acne, and hair loss, and it has also been found to be deficient in some people with eczema.

Dry skin, hair, and nails have been associated with GLA deficiency. According to Nicholas J. Smeh, M.S., author of *Health Risks in Today's Cosmetics*, the EFA linoleic acid, present in many cold-pressed vegetable oils, walnuts, and seeds, was found to be one of the most valuable ingredients in cosmetics by German scientists, because it can help the skin retain moisture and at the same time inhibit acne. Most EFAs are anti-inflammatory. Fish-oil supplements even reduced sunburning in four studies. Fish oil and GLA from evening primrose and borage oil appear to have the most direct anti-inflammatory effects of the EFAs. Keep in mind that many of these studies showing such benefits from supplementation involved individuals who used up to 10 grams (large capsules) of EFAs per day over a few months.

Essential Oils and Other Natural Antimicrobials

Virtually all essential oils (not to be confused with EFAs) have been shown to be antimicrobial to widely varying degrees. Unlike topical or internal antibiotics, none of these antimicrobials has been found to create antibiotic-resistant bacteria. The properties of biblically honored substances such as myrrh, cinnamon, and olive oil are proving their many applications in modern science. Neem, for example, is a unique oil that has been found to be antifungal and antimicrobial when applied topically or orally. (See chapter 12 and the chart at the end of this chapter for other essential oils and their applications.)

There are a number of other natural substances that have antibacterial benefits without the risks associated with commonly prescribed topical or oral antibiotics. Azelaic acid, for example, is a naturally occurring compound from certain grains with some fascinating properties. It is sometimes prescribed instead of topical antibiotics for acne and rosacea. It has also been proven effective in fading the dark patches of melasma, as it has an exfoliating and lightening effect. Zinc as a supplement has been found to have antimicrobial action that is effective against inflamed acne.

Phototherapies

Concentrations of different light wavelengths to treat skin and other problems can be viewed as another form of "nature in therapeutic doses." Also know as phototherapy, these treatments are now successfully being used to treat broken capillaries and redness, acne, sun damage, scars, and more, often replacing harsher methods or drugs. Intense Pulsed Light (IPL) is a breakthrough example of how increasingly effective and gentle light treatments can be, without the possible scarring, discoloration, or downtime associated with lasers. If you have severe skin issues, such treatments make a great jumpstart to your new skin and lifestyle approach, but never a replacement.

Always do some research before deciding on one of these treatments. The options are changing every day. But avoid relying on these procedures to maintain your skin. Don't allow their surface results to distract you from how you treat yourself every day. Aim to glow on your own.

Color Cosmetics

Color cosmetics are the final frontier of nontoxic beauty products. For many years, my professional makeup kit was stocked with all kinds of synthetic concoctions that I used on photo shoots even though I was using natural makeup products on myself. While my pure and potent skin-care discoveries usually went over big with models and celebrities, I couldn't have gotten away with using the aesthetically challenged offerings of nontoxic cosmetics available then. Knowing the safety and sensitivity concerns of coal-tar colors, the irritating nature of perfumes, the dangers of talc inhalation, and the pore-clogging tendencies of mineral oil, I was frustrated with the lack of sophistication and appeal when it came to natural-color cosmetics. But now I'm excited to report that the availability of high-end textures, colors, and even packaging for truly pure cosmetics has improved dramatically in recent years. Even the colors of the mineral-based foundations are now available in the wide range of global, gold-tinged shades that makeup artists seek. There are now beautiful, highly saturated, and finely textured eyeshadows, ultra-hip glosses, and smudgy pencils in must-have colors, minus the petrochemicals, perfumes, preservatives, and coal-tar dyes. You can finally bring both your aesthetic desires and your desire for purity together when it comes to makeup.

Mineral Cosmetics Can Calm Irritated and Post-Treatment Skin

For those with allergy-prone, laser-treated, or otherwise challenged skin or those who simply want to minimize the possible sensitizing factors and inherent toxic risks of conventional color cosmetics, micronized mineral cosmetics are the best answer. Powdered mineral foundations, blushes, and eye shadows, which are colored primarily by iron oxides, actually calm irritation, due to their titanium dioxide and zinc oxides, which are anti-inflammatories. Because they don't contain synthetic dyes, even the lip pencils and blushes can be used in the eye area. Mineral makeup is recommended by dermatologists and plastic surgeons for use after a peel and as the first makeup usable after laser treatment. They provide broad-spectrum UVA and UVB sun protection (usually an FDA-approved SPF 17–20), which can spare sensitive facial skin the added burden and step of applying common sunscreen products. They are also water-resistant but not pore-clogging. The microscopic crystals overlap, allowing the skin to breathe, but they don't crease or accentuate wrinkles as talc-based powders do. Because of the level of coverage, the loose and pressed formulas stand in for liquid foundation and powder without the buildup or cakiness of crème-to-powder foundations. See the Resources for some of my favorites.

> ## *The work associated with high-maintenance skin regimens seems necessary but may be in vain if the true cause of the problem is not being addressed.*

broaden your view of your skin issues

Consider the following chart a symposium of collected science and varied expert opinion on specific skin issues, from conventional to alternative and from medical to nutritional to practical. It includes what is often recommended, overlooked, proven, and observed by doctors, researchers, and experts in specific areas of concern with regard to common skin issues. I've also included some practical lifestyle strategies I have developed and collected. My purpose is to add to what you already know with some additional considerations in your pursuit of real resolutions to your skin issues.

Most of the products in the chart are available at natural-product stores. Ordering information for hard to find products is listed in the Resources.

Note: This chart—as is all of the information in this book—is for educational purposes only. Always seek the guidance of your doctor before starting any supplement regimen or when treating any ailment or condition. As with any therapy, use extra caution if you are pregnant.

SKIN STRATEGY MAKEOVER

BEAUTY-RISKING CHOICE	BEAUTY-SUPPORTING CHOICE	HOLISTIC CONSIDERATIONS
ACNE *(See also Oily Skin)*		
Benzoyl peroxide: Drying and peeling regimens like benzoyl peroxide and vitamin A derivatives can destroy the beauty of the skin and compromise its protective and antiaging matrix. **Tetracycline:** Prescribed for moderate acne, this drug can cause photosensitivity, chronic yeast overgrowth, and digestive problems. **Accutane:** The drug of choice for severe acne can cause dryness of the skin, nose, mouth, lips, and vagina; itching and peeling of the palms and soles; and high cholesterol. Less common side effects include thinning hair, decreased libido, body aches, and liver damage.	**Phospholipids** help restore the acid balance that fights bacteria in the skin. **Azelaic Acid,** a natural compound sometimes prescribed (as Azelex) instead of topical antibiotics, has been shown to have effects comparable to topical benzoyl peroxide gel 5%, tretinoin cream 0.05%, erythromycin cream 2%, and oral tetracycline 0.5 to 1 g/day in treating mild to moderate inflammatory acne. **Tea tree oil** has an effect similar to benzoyl peroxide 5% without making the skin flaky. Tea tree oil and salicylic acid "zit sticks" are a good option for mild acne. **Essential oils** can purify and normalize skin oil. **Neem oil** is antimicrobial and antifungal. **Neroli oil** is purifying and normalizes oil production.	*Excess oil, **skin-cell buildup**, **bacteria**, and **inflammation*** are the issues here. Excess oil production is often hormonal or stress-induced. **Contact reactions** to skin and hair products, phones, and fabrics and many **prescription drugs,** such as steroid inhalers, can contribute to acne. **Food allergies,** iodine-containing foods, and poor digestion or imbalance of intestinal flora can contribute to acne. **Digestive enzymes** and the **probiotic** measures outlined on page 166 can increase the skin's resistance to bacteria and improve digestive issues that might otherwise aggravate acne. **Hydration** is a basic defense against acne, so drink plenty of pure water.

BEAUTY-RISKING CHOICE	BEAUTY-SUPPORTING CHOICE	HOLISTIC CONSIDERATIONS
	Zinc gluconate supplements work comparably to the antibiotic minocycline hydrochloride against inflamed acne, as shown in one double-blind clinical trial.	*Detox measures*, such as green juices, chlorella, milk thistle, turmeric, green tea, red clove, and plant sterolins help the liver and reduce the detox burden on the skin.
	MSM, available in topical products or supplements, is a better utilized form of sulfur that inhibits bacteria and promotes healing.	The low-fiber, high-sugar, and hydrogenated-fat Western diet may be to blame for some acne. In one study, *high fiber intake* reduced inflammatory skin lesions.
	Alpha-lipoic acid topicals can help normalize oil production and shrink pore size, according to Dr. Perricone.	Elevated levels of the androgen hormone DHT—or sensitivity to it—are linked to some forms of treatment-resistant acne, according to the New Zealand Dermatological Society. Saw palmetto berry extract is known to block DHT.
	Phototherapy: Recent studies in the U.K. suggest isolated *red- and blue-light wavelengths* can help mild to moderate acne by killing bacteria and reducing inflammation.	
	Cold-water fish, fish oil, or evening-primrose supplements have hormone-balancing and anti-inflammatory effects.	

BEAUTY-RISKING CHOICE	BEAUTY-SUPPORTING CHOICE	HOLISTIC CONSIDERATIONS
DANDRUFF		
Resorcinol found in dandruff shampoos can cause discoloration and dermatitis. *Coal tar–containing shampoos* can irritate the scalp and may be toxic.	*Pyrithione Zinc* (available in shampoos) alleviated dandruff in a recent study. *Tea tree oil*–containing hair cleansers, free of SLS, can provide antifungal action without irritation. *Antifungal, antimicrobial substances* like oregano oil, grapefruit seed extract (GSE), and tea tree oil added to scalp preparations in small amounts may help. *Apple-cider vinegar* normalizes scalp pH, which can help inhibit bacteria and fungus.	First rule out the simplest cause of flakes and irritation, which might be your *hair products*. See what happens if you change them. *Dry scalp* flakes may accompany dry skin and fungal or inflammatory skin and body conditions (see "Inflammatory Skin Problems" for dietary considerations). *GLA* supplements may help dry scalp and inflammation.
DARK SPOTS OR PATCHES		
Skin lighteners containing hydroquinone can cause skin discoloration and allergic reactions. Hydroquinone is made from crystalline phenol, a suspected carcinogen. *Lasers* do not perform well on melasma discolorations, according to Dr. Deborah Jaliman, a New York City dermatologist.	*Azelaic acid* is an effective and safer bleaching agent. Some data suggest that topical azelaic acid, used twice daily with a broad-spectrum sunscreen, works as well as hydroquinone 4% creams. *Kojic acid* inhibits melanin. Vitamin C, licorice, and bioflavanoids can lighten the skin somewhat.	*Hormonal changes,* such as those associated with pregnancy or use of birth-control pills, often contribute to dark spots and patches or melasma— the "mask of pregnancy." This can only be avoided by vigilantly *protecting your skin from sun exposure.* Use mineral-based sunscreens for maximum, safe protection.

BEAUTY-RISKING CHOICE	BEAUTY-SUPPORTING CHOICE	HOLISTIC CONSIDERATIONS
DARK SPOTS OR PATCHES (continued)		
	Skin Answer contains glycoalkaloids, which actually exfoliate raised, rough spots and patches of sun-damaged skin in four to six weeks.	*Mineral makeup* gives sun protection, anti-inflammatory benefits, and aesthetic coverage without irritation.
	Lasers and microdermabrasion: For brown spots that go with sun damage, Dr. Jaliman recommends versa pulse laser. She recommends microdermabrasion for melasma.	*Antioxidants* taken internally and applied to the skin can offer added protection from sun.
DRY LIPS		
Phenol-containing mineral oil or petrolatum-based lip balms cause skin irritation, dryness, and "lip balm addiction."	*Skin-compatible oils and lip balms* containing ingredients like shea butter cocoa butter, coconut oil, beeswax, calendula, aloe, allantoin (comfrey root), and vitamins C and E all truly hydrate, heal, and protect the lips, not just seal them.	*Avoid contact with water* in the colder months. Try applying lip balm *before* you brush your teeth if your lips are chapped.
		Avoid irritating and drying products such as alcohol-containing mouthwashes and SLS-containing toothpastes.

BEAUTY-RISKING CHOICE	BEAUTY-SUPPORTING CHOICE	HOLISTIC CONSIDERATIONS
DRY SKIN		
Foaming and detergent cleansers, soaps, and bubble baths make dry skin worse. Dermatologist-recommended *propylene glycol–based cleansers* can still irritate and dry the skin. *Mineral oil and petrolatum-based* body moisturizers, body oil, baby oil, bath oil, and lip balms can actually leave the skin and lips dryer.	*Cleansing milks and non-stripping cleansers* free of irritants like propylene glycol and detergents help your skin recover its own protection. *Phospholipids* and *GLA-containing moisturizers and supplements* can rebuild the lipid barrier that prevents dry rough skin. *Skin-compatible oils* such as jojoba, sweet almond oil, apricot kernel oil, primrose oil, avocado, azulene, squalane, emu oil, neem, olive oil, hemp oil, and sesame oil contain fatty acids that work in concert with sebum rather than against it or blocking it, like mineral oil. *Injuv* is a new supplement that may increase the level of hyaluronic acid in the body. Hyaluronic acid acts as a sponge, holding moisture within the skin. (More studies need to be done on this supplement.)	A *humidifier* will help alleviate dryness. Increased *water intake* and decreased caffeine and alcohol intake can help. Dry skin, along with brittle hair, sparse eyebrows, or sensitivity to cold, are common symptoms of *thyroid issues*. *Chlorinated water* can contribute to dry skin. *Installing a shower filter* can make an unbelievable difference.

BEAUTY-RISKING CHOICE	BEAUTY-SUPPORTING CHOICE	HOLISTIC CONSIDERATIONS

INFLAMMATORY SKIN PROBLEMS
(See also Sensitive Skin, Dry Skin, and Dandruff)

Steroid ointments used over prolonged periods thin the skin and compromise its basic immunity, making recurrences more likely and often worse.	*Pyrithione Zinc* 0.2% sprays, lotions, and shampoos have shown remarkable efficacy for clearing up psoriasis and similar conditions.	*There are countless causes for dermatitis.* Rule out contact allergens first. For the best possible outcome, pay close attention to what triggers your symptoms.
Coal-tar preparations can cause sun sensitivity and irritation.	*Long-term use of both licorice* (Glycyrrhiza glabra) and *German Camillosan chamomile* have been shown to be comparable in effect to long-term topical hydrocortisone treatments in inflammatory skin conditions.	*Allergies, food sensitivities, and digestive problems* are strongly linked with certain types of eczema and psoriasis. Test for food sensitivities or try an elimination diet.
Heavy petrolatum or mineral oil-based creams can ultimately inhibit the skin's healing function.		*Compromised protein digestion and auto-immune flare-ups* may be linked with psoriasis, according to Michael T. Murray, N.D., author of *Natural Alternatives to Over-the-Counter and Prescription Drugs.*
Psoriasis treatments like UVB and narrow-band UVB work on psoriasis but can raise issues of sun damage and skin cancer.	*Healing botanicals* like aloe and allantoin (comfrey) can reduce discomfort and speed healing.	
PUVA, which involves the use of Psoralens, a photo-sensitizing drug, plus UVA light exposure, has been found to be more effective than UVB but carries skin-cancer risks.	*Capsaicin* (hot pepper) cream reduced psoriasis scaling and redness significantly when using capsaicin .025 cream four times a day for six weeks.	*Increased fiber intake* and *decreased sugar intake* (the antifungal diet) decreased seborrheic eczema in one study.
	Climatotherapy for psoriasis is a treatment given only at the Dead Sea clinics in Israel that includes liberal sunlight exposure and bathing in the Dead Sea. In one study, it produced a clearing of 80 to 100 percent in 88 percent of over 1,000 patients treated.	The *probiotic* measures on page 166 may help reduce the digestive and inflammatory issues that can lead to some types of eczema and psoriasis flair-ups.

BEAUTY-RISKING CHOICE	BEAUTY-SUPPORTING CHOICE	HOLISTIC CONSIDERATIONS
INFLAMMATORY SKIN PROBLEMS (continued)		
	Mahonia aquifolium, or *Oregon-grape root* improved psoriasis symptoms in sufferers over twelve weeks in a large-scale German study and has also been shown to work on eczema. Low pH **water** has antimicrobial properties and may benefit inflammatory skin conditions. A small device called Charme™ delivers fresh, low pH water without the large machinery previously required.	*EFAs*, particularly *GLA* from borage and evening-primrose oil, and EPA from fish, have been found to help inflammatory skin disorders. Four to 10 grams per day have been used by individuals in most studies. *Anti-inflammatory supplements*, like MSM, nettle, milk thistle, green tea, and turmeric may help.
OILY SKIN		
Soaps and other foaming or detergent cleansers and alcohol-based astringents and products that leave the skin tight cause oily rebound and strip the skin's acid mantle protection.	*Essential oil blends* and moisturizers that include neem, ylang ylang, neroli, and lavender can purify the skin and normalize oil production.	*If you have oily skin* you will have fewer wrinkles as you age. See also *EFAs* and *alpha-lipoic acid* under "Acne."

BEAUTY-RISKING CHOICE	BEAUTY-SUPPORTING CHOICE	HOLISTIC CONSIDERATIONS
ROSACEA AND BROKEN CAPILLARIES *(See also Inflammatory Skin Problems)*		
The characteristic redness, broken capillaries, and sometimes acne associated with rosacea is commonly treated with topical antibiotics.	**Azelaic Acid** is sometimes used or prescribed (as Azelex) instead of topical antibiotics but does not cause resistant bacteria to develop.	With rosacea, it's largely about *avoiding the triggers*, such as alcohol, hot drinks, and spicy foods.
See **Accutane** cautions under "Acne."	**Vitamin K** and horse-chestnut creams may strengthen weakened capillaries.	In *Natural Alternatives to Over-the-Counter and Prescription Drugs*, Michael T. Murray, N.D., points to *hydrochloric acid (HCL) deficiency* as a possible culprit in some cases of rosacea. Early science supports this.
Steroids can actually cause rosacea and broken capillaries by thinning the skin and weakening capillary walls.	**Demodicidin** is a soap that may kill both the Folliculorum and Brevis types of Demodex human associated with acne rosacea.	According to Arlen Brownstein, M.S., N.D., and Donna Schoemaker, C.N., authors of *Rosacea: Your Self-Help Guide*, drinking liquids with meals can dilute digestive enzymes that break down protein.
Conventional cosmetics used to cover rosacea can irritate the condition by causing photo-sensitivity and acne.	**Strontium-containing products** have been shown to reduce sensitivity to skin products.	*Leaky gut*, a condition in which lack of good bacteria causes increased intestinal-wall permeability, may worsen inflammatory skin issues (see also "Acne" and "Inflammatory Skin Problems") and consider the probiotic measures on page 166.
Avoid any skin products containing *solvents, alcohol, abrasives,* or *exfoliants.* Eliminate common irritants, such as perfume (see "Sensitive Skin").	**Blue-light therapy** may help acne rosacea.	*Mineral cosmetics* achieve good coverage and sun protection while avoiding the irritation of synthetic color cosmetics and sunscreens.
	Intense Pulsed Light Therapy (IPL, or Photo-Derm) has been proven effective for treatment of rosacea and may even work for some people who don't respond to laser treatments while sparing them the possible permanent side effects and the downtime of laser treatments.	

BEAUTY-RISKING CHOICE	BEAUTY-SUPPORTING CHOICE	HOLISTIC CONSIDERATIONS
SCARS		
Erbium and carbon-dioxide laser treatments can be effective for acne scars and other scars but can cause further scarring and pigmentation problems, particularly for people with medium and dark skin tones and requires downtime. (It works better for fair skin, according to Dr. Jaliman.)	*Topical silicone gels* can reduce and flatten some raised scars over months of use. Works best with new scars. According to Dr. Perricone, *alpha-lipoic acid* can prevent and reverse scar formation. *Laser and light therapies:* For shallow acne scars, Dr. Jaliman recommends the *Cool Touch II laser* for any skin color (caveat: treatments may take over five months). For deeper scars, she recommends various combinations of punch-grafting, fillers (such as collagen and hyaluronic acid), and microdermabrasion.	*Sunlight* on traumatized skin or even a healing pimple can leave a dark spot, particularly during hormonal fluctuations, so keep sunlight off any skin blemish. A *spray-on mineral-based sunscreen* gives better overall protection, allows the skin to breathe, and is anti-inflammatory and delicate to apply. *Keeping a wound clean* is important. A topical spray containing citrus-seed extract offers effective antimicrobial action to prevent additional scarring. Picking at skin or scabs can cause scarring.
SENSITIVE SKIN (See also Inflammatory Skin Problems)		
Harsh skin products that contain solvents, fragrances, detergents, and high levels of preservatives sensitize the skin.	*Naturally scented and formulated products* with preservatives listed last on the ingredients list or not at all may cause less irritation.	*Cosmetic* and *contact irritants* can sensitize and irritate the skin.

BEAUTY-RISKING CHOICE	BEAUTY-SUPPORTING CHOICE	HOLISTIC CONSIDERATIONS

SENSITIVE SKIN (continued)

BEAUTY-RISKING CHOICE	BEAUTY-SUPPORTING CHOICE	HOLISTIC CONSIDERATIONS
Foaming bath products, fragranced laundry detergent, and *fabric softeners* can also sensitize and irritate the skin.	*Phospholipid-*containing moisturizers can help restore the barrier that keeps irritants from penetrating the skin.	*Perfume* and *nail-polish ingredients* like formaldehyde and toluene are strong sensitizers.
AHAs and other irritating exfoliants can sensitize the skin by compromising its natural barrier to irritants.	*Strontium-*containing skin products can inhibit the sensitization from cosmetic ingredients and related dermatitis.	*Formaldehyde* can also be on new clothes, sheets, or towels and can set off a reaction that can leave you sensitized for weeks.
Conventional color cosmetics contain known irritants, like coal-tar dyes and perfumes.	*Use mineral-based color cosmetics* and cosmetics free of perfumes, petro-chemicals, and preservatives.	*Nickel* in fashion jewelry, car-key chains, eyeglasses and zippers can sensitize skin and cause rashes.
Dr. Jaliman often observes skin reactions from *nail polish, nail adhesives, hair color, mascara,* and eye crops containing the preservative *thimerosol. Soaps, shampoos, contact-lens solutions* and *eye-makeup removers* containing the preservative *Cat-B* can all cause redness and skin flakes.	*Kinetin (or Kinerase)* is a plant-derived substance that has been shown in some studies to effectively diminish wrinkles without irritation.	*An imbalance in body ecology* can make the skin more reactive. See "Pro-Beauty Probiotics" on page 166 for measures that may help.
	Colloidal oatmeal and *Dead Sea salts* in the bath can bring substantial relief of irritation.	*Prescription drugs* can sensitize the skin.

VARICOSE AND SPIDER VEINS

BEAUTY-RISKING CHOICE	BEAUTY-SUPPORTING CHOICE	HOLISTIC CONSIDERATIONS
Compression hose therapy for varicose veins is uncomfortable, hygienically unsmart, and doesn't address the real cause and dangers of varicose veins.	*Horse-chestnut-seed extract* has been shown to be comparable to compression hose therapy in decreasing ankle circumference and reducing the swelling of varicose veins.	*Pregnancy, sitting cross-legged,* and *constipation* are believed to contribute to varicose veins. Keeping legs elevated when possible (especially while sleeping) helps reduce swelling.

VARICOSE AND SPIDER VEINS (continued)

BEAUTY-RISKING CHOICE	BEAUTY-SUPPORTING CHOICE	HOLISTIC CONSIDERATIONS
Laser procedures can work, but they tend to be expensive and results are temporary, leaving the health issue unresolved.	cose veins in women with chronic venous insufficiency. Other natural varicose vein remedies, such as the bioflavanoid rutin, work, but horse-chestnut-seed extract was shown to be five hundred times more effective. *Vitamin K* is a proven coagulant that minimizes bruising and is widely used by dermatologists to minimize and strengthen broken capillaries. *Sclerotherapy, lasers, stripping:* According to Dr. Jaliman, it's hard to know which procedure works best on an individual's veins until you try them. Sclerotherapy injects a chemical into varicose veins that damages and collapses the vein (the bloodflow is safely rerouted). Deep-set veins and spider veins respond well to the *Lira Laser*, which penetrates the skin without irritating it. Bulging varicose veins may need to be "stripped out."	Cultures with *diets low in refined foods* rarely suffer from varicose veins. *Address vein problems as health issues:* If you use laser, schlerotherapy, or stripping techniques, use them as a jump start, but take steps to address the cause of the veins, which may signal trouble throughout the body. Horse-chestnut-seed extract, for example, strengthens the vasculature throughout the body rather than offering only a cosmetic effect. Food and beverage upgrades, supplements, and exercise may help you diminish or avoid a recurrence of the veins.

BEAUTY-RISKING CHOICE	BEAUTY-SUPPORTING CHOICE	HOLISTIC CONSIDERATIONS

WRINKLES

See "Dry Skin" for skin products to avoid.

Alpha-hydroxy acids (AHAs): Long-term alpha- and beta-hydroxy and glycolic acid use or abuse can make skin irritated, dry, tight, thin, and raw or dull. It also causes makeup to look blotchy.

Long-term effects of AHAs, BHAs, regular lasering and peels, and any other types of perpetual irritation and accelerated exfoliation are unknown.

Retin-A or **Renova:** Prescribed for their wrinkle- and acne-reducing peeling action that increases cell turnover, these synthetic vitamin A derivatives can be extremely irritating and leave the skin red and flaky. They a so leave the skin intensely vulnerable to the sun, water loss, and offending substances that are more likely to be absorbed by the skin after treatment.

Phospholipids can rebuild the hydrolipid barrier and prevent premature aging of the skin.

Studies have proven that high-potency topically-applied vitamin C serums can rebuild collagen.

According to Dr. Perricone, the C-ester form of vitamin C works without the irritation caused by the L-ascorbic acid form of vitamin C. He recommends **vitamin C-ester serums** in combination with **DMAE** and **alpha-lipoic acid** to reverse wrinkles and lift the face.

See **Kinetin** under "Sensitive Skin."

Marine lipids and extracts, **papaya enzymes,** and **licorice-containing moisturizers** soften and stimulate skin renewal without irritation.

The anti-glycation supplements or topicals containing **carnosine** may inhibit the cross-linking that causes wrinkles.

See **Injuv** under "Dry Skin."

Smoking, too much **sun** and **sugar, compromised skin barrier** due to harsh products, fat or **EFA deficiency** in the diet all contribute to wrinkles.

Wrinkle alert: If you smoke, you are two to three times more likely to have moderate to severe wrinkles at age forty or older than a nonsmoker.

GLA supplements help to rebuild the skin's barrier from moisture evaporation and help prevent premature skin aging due to water loss.

Eating sugar and **high-glycemic foods** induces glycation as well as collagen cross-linking that causes wrinkles. **Alpha-lipoic acid** inhibits the glycation process.

Wrinkle-fighting antioxidants that inhibit skin damage and aging: **vitamins C, E (d-alpha tocopherol),** and **A, beta carotene, alpha-lipoic acid, melotonin, pycnogenol, superoxide dismutase (S.O.D.), antioxidant-rich fruits and vegetables, green tea, grapeseed extract,** and **CoQ10.**

BEAUTY-RISKING CHOICE	BEAUTY-SUPPORTING CHOICE	HOLISTIC CONSIDERATIONS
WRINKLES (continued)		
	Light therapy: For crinkles and crepiness, Dr. Jaliman recommends the Cool Touch laser. Starting a new regimen of collagen-building supplements, serums, and sun-protective measures at the same time will help you glow on your own so you won't need to depend on long-term treatments. *Toki collagen drink* has been shown to increase collagen levels in the blood, and anecdotal evidence is compelling for its effects in plumping up the skin.	*Vitamin E* has been proven to protect the skin from sun damage. Related vitamin E substances called *tocotrienols* may provide even more potent protection. *Vitamin A* increases cell turnover and hydration and diminishes wrinkles.

anatomy of a holistic beauty splurge

Take a busy woman with dry skin and $125 or so to spend on her seasonal beauty splurge. Before reading this book, she might have splurged on the latest department-store skin regimen with "token" botanicals or patented ingredients in a base of cheap carriers and known irritants. Now, with the same $125, she could start with a $45 vitamin C serum, buy a shower filter for $65, upgrade her current body soap to one of pure olive oil for $2, and buy a bottle of fish-oil capsules for $12. With this new regimen she may very well eliminate her dry, itchy skin and her need for heavy lotions and creams forever while improving her overall health in ways that will continue to unfold in the months and even years to come. She is now light-years beyond what any fancy dry-skin regimen will ever deliver. The degree to which our beauty splurges can truly transform us is limited only by our knowledge of the options.

what remains between you and your best glow

Now that you've begun to consider the deeper issues behind your skin challenges, you have new clues to direct your own process of shedding and to cultivate your best glow. In the following chapters, you'll learn how to weed out and shed even more chemical and emotional wild cards that stand between you and your most radiant potential.

the BATHROOM-CABINET MAKEOVER

Treating minor day-to-day discomforts and irritations with quick fixes that address only your symptoms while imposing new burdens on the body can be a drain on the energy that could otherwise be making life—and you—beautiful. Planning and implementing your own bathroom-cabinet makeover to maximize and expand your rewards while minimizing the risks is one of the most exciting ways to engage your self-respect and self-preservation instincts.

the bathroom-cabinet makeover chart

Here is just a small sample of the kinds of real rewards you can get from a new class of bathroom cabinet staples. These products can get you away from quick fixes and don't cause side effects. Once known only to holistic connoisseurs who did their homework, these now-proven alternatives may spare you untold assaults. As in every area of pro-beauty upgrades, each prevented assault will be beauty in the bank.

Again, the following chart is for educational purposes only and is not intended to diagnose or treat illnesses. If you are taking prescription medications or specific over-the-counter regimens recommended by your doctor, don't discontinue them on your own. Enlist your doctor's supervision and tell him or her what alternatives you'd like to consider. Your doctor may or may not be familiar with some of the products and options listed here and throughout this book, but he or she should be responsive to the published studies listed in the bibliography that correspond with the substances listed in the following charts. If your doctor is not amenable to talking about incorporating nondrug approaches, see "Organizations, Educational Resources, and Services" in the Resources to find a doctor near you who integrates both conventional and alternative approaches. Such a move could greatly improve the future of your beauty.

Although I've chosen to address only a small sampling of common products and safe, science-backed alternatives that you and your doctor can incorporate, I heartily encourage you to apply the same discerning principles to evaluate every single product on your shelves: read what your products contain, what side effects they may have (remember that long-term side effects aren't always listed on labels), and consider any alternatives that may serve you better.

These products can get you away from quick fixes and don't cause side effects.

ALLERGY AND SINUS PRODUCTS

BEAUTY-RISKING CHOICE	PRO-BEAUTY ALTERNATIVES	HOLISTIC CONSIDERATIONS
Most prescription *antihistamines* can cause dry mouth, dry nose, headache, and sleep problems.	*Nasalcrom, a homeopathic nasal spray,* contains cromolyn sodium, proven to both prevent and reduce nasal allergy symptoms with no side effects.	Just as *fish oil* reduces some allergic skin conditions, it also reduces allergies and asthma symptoms.
Most *nasal sprays* can cause swelling of nasal tissue. In addition, they are not safe for those with high blood pressure.	*The xylitol-containing nasal spray called Xlear* has been shown to inhibit bacteria, including the bacteria that can cause ear infections, by an anti-adherence action thought to be similar to how cranberry works in the urinary tract.	Other *anti-inflammatory supplements* that help both nasal and skin allergies are stinging nettle, vitamin C, magnesium, and the bioflavanoid quercitin, which is a natural histamine suppressor.
Long-term side effects of *steroid drugs and inhalers* range from the unsightly to serious, including bone loss, "moon face," blood-sugar imbalances, Dowager's hump, bloated abdomen, and acne (particularly around the chin). Immunity also is compromised, leaving you more open to infections.	*Zinc-based nasal gel (Zicam)* has been proven to stop sinus infections in their tracks and reduce the duration of the common cold without side effects.	*Douching nasal passages* with salt water from your hands or a porcelain nasal cup can curtail sinus infections (if you can stand the process of snorting water through one nostril). *Saline nasal sprays* work in a similar way without the hassle.
Always consult your physician before discontinuing any kind of steroid, allergy, or asthma medication. That said, you may consider it worthwhile to look into ways to reduce your need for these kinds of medications.	*Saline sprays* such as Ocean keep nasal passages moist and cleansed.	A holistic health practitioner can help you identify food sensitivities and incorporate *supplements* which may reduce *digestive issues* that can affect your allergies.

BEAUTY-RISKING CHOICE	PRO-BEAUTY ALTERNATIVES	HOLISTIC CONSIDERATIONS
ANTIPERSPIRANTS AND DEODORANTS		
Aluminum chlorohydrate: The man-made form of aluminum, which is contained in antiperspirants, is suspected by many scientists to accumulate in tissues, particularly when applied to broken skin. *Conventional deodorants that do not contain aluminum* tend to be highly perfumed and contain petrochemicals. Given what we are starting to learn about the accumulation of chemicals in the body, applying them over broken skin may not be a great idea.	*Natural deodorants containing antimicrobial ingredients* like tea tree oil, coriander, and GSE are getting more effective. Trial and error is the best way to find what works with your chemistry. *Lavilin* is one of the strongest natural deodorants. Caveat: It's expensive.	*Internal deodorants* containing body deodorizers like chlorophyll and activated charcoal have hit the market. All sorts of factors are responsible for our scent, so these products may or may not work for you. Detoxifying and keeping your pipes clean with *fiber, greens,* my *Beauty Detox Elixir* (see chapter 5), *liver-supportive* and *probiotic supplements,* and lots of water is the best way to usher out waste that could otherwise putrify in the digestive tract and even affect your breath.
COLD-SORE PRODUCTS		
Valtrex, Zovirax, and *Famvir* take several days to work and often fail, especially on acyclovir (Zovirax)-resistant strains of the herpes virus. *Prescription antiviral* pills may cause headache, nausea, and diarrhea.	*ViraMedx®* is the first topical treatment proven to stop the virus that causes herpes and give substantial and consistent healing in about twenty-four hours (other treatments take five to ten days). It is less expensive, and because of the nature of its mechanism of action, is effective on acyclovir-resistant strains of herpes and less likely to cause them to mutate into drug-resistant strains.	*Sun, stress,* and *illness* can bring on cold sore outbreaks, so do all you can to support your immunity. The amino acid *L-arginine* from any source, including nuts, can aggravate herpes, while the amino acid *L-lysine* may help prevent outbreaks.

BEAUTY-RISKING CHOICE	PRO-BEAUTY ALTERNATIVES	HOLISTIC CONSIDERATIONS

COLD-SORE PRODUCTS (continued)

BEAUTY-RISKING CHOICE	PRO-BEAUTY ALTERNATIVES	HOLISTIC CONSIDERATIONS
	Tea tree oil treated cold sores comparably to acyclovir 5% in one randomized, placebo-controlled pilot study.	*Green and black tea,* even in moderate amounts, has been shown to deactivate E. coli and herpes simplex types I and II virus in the mouth.
		Herpanacine and *Herpilyn* are both supplements that inhibit herpes outbreaks.

HAIR-LOSS PRODUCTS

BEAUTY-RISKING CHOICE	PRO-BEAUTY ALTERNATIVES	HOLISTIC CONSIDERATIONS
Minoxidil (Rogaine): Common side effects are mainly scalp irritation or itching, though researchers at the University of Toronto found that long-term use can lead to heart changes.	Natural *DHT-blocking hair-loss preparations* have actions similar to Propecia without the side effects.	*Sluggish thyroid function, trauma, surgery, stress,* and *heredity* all contribute to hair loss.
Propecia (finasteride) can throw off PSA-test results, cause loss of libido or erectile dysfunction in some men, and cannot be taken by women because of concerns over possible birth defects.	*Hair Genesis,* a nondrug formula containing the DHL-blocker saw palmetto berry and plant sterols, was shown in a recent double-blind, placebo-controlled study to be a viable, safer alternative to prescription hair-loss drugs.	*Key nutrients* for healthier hair: *MSM* (sulfur), *silica*, *EFAs, vitamin B* (biotin, pantathenic acid, and inositol).
	A natural hair-loss product called *Viviscal* has shown significant clinical effectiveness against several types of hair loss, including alopecia areata, a type of hair loss thought to be stress- or autoimmune-related.	*L-arginine*'s ability to boost nitric oxide, which relaxes and dilates the hair follicle, along with its established circulatory effects (it is often included in "herbal Viagra" and creams that bring circulation to the hands and feet) and ability to aid the release of hGH make it a logical topical and internal ingredient in hair formulas.

BEAUTY-RISKING CHOICE	PRO-BEAUTY ALTERNATIVES	HOLISTIC CONSIDERATIONS
HAIR-LOSS PRODUCTS (continued)		
	Nitric oxide (NO) and related compounds or precursors are important to hair-follicle health since they relax the hair follicle, working in a similar way to minoxidil. Dr. Peter Proctor, a noted hair-loss researcher who holds several patents for hair-loss treatments, developed hair formulas based on a nitro compound called *NANO (3-carboxylic acid pyridine-N-oxide)*, which he refers to as "natural minoxidil." In one double-blind trial, an *essential oil combination of rosemary, lavender, thyme,* and *cedarwood* (a few drops each) mixed with a jojoba and grapeseed-oil carrier combination (20mL) sped regrowth of hair. The essential oils were thought to block the autoimmune reaction that caused the hair loss.	*Shen Min* is an herbal compound based on the Chinese medicinal herb *he shou wu*, or *fo-ti*, used traditionally to prevent hair loss and graying and aging in general. There has been no clinical proof yet regarding hair growth (though studies show it lowers cholesterol). *Circulation to the scalp* through exercise and massage are important. *Quality fats* and the *elimination of hydrogenated fats* are crucial to nourishment of the hair follicles and reducing inflammation.
INSECT REPELLENT		
DEET: Frequent and long-term use can cause brain deficits in vulnerable populations, especially children, according to a July 2002 Duke University Heath Note.	*Lemongrass* has been shown to be comparable in effectiveness to many commercial insect repellents in one study.	Taking plenty of *B vitamins* makes you less appealing to mosquitos.

BEAUTY-RISKING CHOICE	PRO-BEAUTY ALTERNATIVES	HOLISTIC CONSIDERATIONS

MOUTH-CARE PRODUCTS

Toothpastes that contain SLS are proven skin and mouth irritants. They are also known to cause canker sores. *Conventional mouthwashes* with an alcohol content of 25 percent have been shown to increase the risk of oral cancers by more than 90 percent. They also dry the mouth, which can cause tooth decay. *Professional teeth whiteners* and home whitening programs are expensive and can contain SLS and other irritants.	*Herbal toothpastes and mouthwashes* without SLS and alcohol can spare you irritation and canker sores and provide a spectrum of far greater benefits with ingredients like aloe, echinacea, goldenseal, neem, TTO, and clove to keep your mouth clean and teeth and gums healthy. *Hydrogen peroxide* (the basis of most expensive teeth-whitening products) made into a paste with baking soda whitens teeth very well and can reverse some gum problems that might otherwise require surgery, according to many dentists. *Sonic toothbrushes* can disinfect the mouth below the gumline and whiten teeth while eliminating some gum infections and stopping some types of canker sores in their tracks. *Xylitol-containing gum and oral-care products* can protect teeth from bacteria. This natural birch sugar inhibited bacteria, including streptococci and plaque, in clinical trials. It also aids in the remineralization of tooth enamel.	*Avoiding mouth infections* is important to maintaining fresh breath and also affects your overall health. Supplements like *CoQ10* and *grapeseed extract* have been shown to improve gum health. *Oolong tea* reduces plaque deposits on teeth. *Green and black tea,* even in moderate amounts, have recently been shown in preliminary studies to inhibit the bacteria that causes tooth decay and even deactivated E. coli and herpes simplex types I and II in the mouth. *Cleaning the tongue* with your toothbrush, a tongue scraper, or a special tongue brush helps.

BEAUTY-RISKING CHOICE	PRO-BEAUTY ALTERNATIVES	HOLISTIC CONSIDERATIONS

NAIL PRODUCTS

BEAUTY-RISKING CHOICE	PRO-BEAUTY ALTERNATIVES	HOLISTIC CONSIDERATIONS
Nail fungus drugs: The prescription anti-fungals **Sporanox** and **Lamisil** are associated with liver toxicity. *Typical nail polishes and strengtheners* only coat the nail to thicken it, which protects the nail from breakage while actually drying out the nail bed and burdening the nail (and your system) with harmful chemicals like **formaldehyde, toluene,** and **dibutyl pthalate.** These ingredients can also cause severe skin rashes.	A double-blind study compared *TTO's* effectiveness against nail fungus to its prescription counterpart, clotrimazole, and showed TTO to be just as effective. To eliminate nail fungus, Dr. Julian Whitaker, editor of the newsletter *Health and Healing*, recommends rubbing the oil onto the nail and adjacent skin twice daily. It may take eight to ten months before the infection is gone. **Myrrh** is a substance that is known to substantially penetrate and strengthen the nails.	*Fungal issues* such as Candida yeast and nail infections can signal systemic yeast overgrowth problems in the digestive tract. *Staying away from sugar and flour* and taking *probiotics* can reduce symptoms and help treatments work better. *Skin, hair, and nail supplements* contain connective tissue–supporting nutrients like sulfur (or its more bio-available form, MSM), silica, B vitamins, and EFAs to create resilient, healthier nails (and hair and skin) in a few months.

SUNSCREEN

BEAUTY-RISKING CHOICE	PRO-BEAUTY ALTERNATIVES	HOLISTIC CONSIDERATIONS
Standard chemical sunscreens: These common chemical sunscreen ingredients have been found in animal studies to accumulate in breast milk and to influence hormonal systems: 4-Methyl-Benzyliden-camphor (4-MBC), Oxybenzone, Benzophenone-3, Octyl-methoxy-cinnamates (OMC), Octyl-Dimethyl-Para-Amino-Benzoic Acid (OD-PABA), and Homosalate (HMS).	*Micronized zinc oxide (Z-cote) and titanium dioxide–based sunscreens:* Titanium dioxide can block both UVA and UVB rays with no known toxicity if used externally. Zinc oxide complements titanium dioxide. The new sprays go on easily and lightly and don't make you white. *Antioxidant ingredients* like vitamins C and E and green tea have been proven to make sunscreens more effective.	*Antioxidant supplements* such as *green tea,* *alpha-lipoic acid,* and *vitamins C* and *E* have been shown to inhibit sun damage and reduce inflammation. There are preliminary studies that have shown a connection between *the quality of fat we eat* and our skin's ability to withstand the sun. *EFAs* have been shown to offer some natural sun protection.

BEAUTY-RISKING CHOICE	PRO-BEAUTY ALTERNATIVES	HOLISTIC CONSIDERATIONS
SUNSCREEN (*continued*)		
	Mineral-based sunscreens not only provide complete protection from the sun but they also have anti-inflammatory effects rather than sensitizing and harming the skin.	
TALC OR BABY POWDER		
Talc has been linked with ovarian cancer. One study showed ovarian cancer risk to be 3.28 times higher in women who used talc in the genital area than for those who didn't. Talc has been discovered in ovarian tumors and in lungs.	*Cornstarch or silk-based powders* are a safer choice, especially for babies!	Whether its you or your baby you're taking care of, you can avoid a myriad of confirmed irritants and toxins by using *natural baby products* instead of standard powders, mineral oil, and baby wipes.

HULDA: CHRONIC DERMATITIS CLEARED UNEXPECTEDLY

Until she attended my seven-day cruise program in November 2000, Hulda had been plagued by hives for a few years. She would get welts over her entire body, especially under her arms and breasts. She had been to several doctors, was given different diagnoses, including shingles, for which she was given Valtrex, and contact dermatitis of unknown origin, for which she was given antihistamines, and finally psoriasis, for which she was prescribed steroid ointments. These prescriptions gave only minimal and temporary relief. She was desperately seeking a solution.

After one of my sessions on cosmetics ingredients, Hulda counted her antiperspirant/deodorant roll-on, which was labeled as hypoallergenic, among one of the products she would phase out of her personal-care routine. She wanted to use a product that would keep her fresh without blocking her normal perspiration. To her complete surprise, she experienced a marked reversal of her hives only a few days after discontinuing the product, and in about two weeks her skin had cleared completely. She now uses a calendula-based deodorant and has never had a recurrence of her problem.

the big guns: new bathroom-cabinet staples to stock

The following is short list of particularly powerful, natural antimicrobials and immune boosters you should know about for occasional times of need. Available through health and vitamin stores, these substances can be used in a wide variety of applications, and with your doctor's supervision, you may even use them to avoid resorting to antibiotics and the cascade of syndromes and skindromes that come with them.

THE BIG GUNS

Echinacea/goldenseal tincture	Echinacea and goldenseal tincture can enhance your resistance when you're under the weather. Echinacea has proven immune-boosting effects, and goldenseal has proven antimicrobial effects.
Grapefruit-seed extract (GSE)	Grapefruit-seed extract (GSE), not to be confused with grapeseed extract, has demonstrated strong antibacterial action against a wide range of nasty bacteria. Ask your doctor if you can try it before resorting to harsher drugs. Available in capsules, liquid, sprays for the skin and feet, foot powders, deodorant, and other products.
Oregano oil	Oregano oil has been shown to destroy Candida albicans yeast both in vitro and in vivo, as well as strep, pneumonia, staphylococcus, and E. coli bacteria in vitro (test tube studies). The oil is strong and can be blended in small amounts into topical preparations. Do not apply to delicate skin. A few drops can be added to water and taken internally. And it's fantastic in cooking!
Tea tree oil (TTO)	The essential oil of melaleuca alternifolia (tea tree), or TTO, has broad-spectrum antimicrobial activity and fights nail fungus, cold sores, and Candida yeast. TTO nasal ointment and body wash has worked against antibiotic-resistant strains of staphylococcus aureus better than conventional antibacterial nasal ointment and antibacterial (trichlosan-containing) soaps. Used in minute amounts, it can be added to scalp, foot, and skin preparations and used in mouth products.
Cranberry capsules	Cranberry helps prevent urinary-tract infections.
Xylitol	Xylitol is an amazing natural sugar found in birch. It can prevent and halt sinus and middle-ear infections and inhibit bacteria by an anti-adherence action. Xylitol-containing gum inhibits teeth and gum infections.

KAREN GETS OFF THE ANTIBIOTIC MERRY-GO-ROUND WITH GSE

After making the connection between her frequent antibiotic use and her chronic digestive problems, Karen decided to try GSE for her yeast infection. With her gynecologist's blessing, she decided to fight her impulse to use antibiotics in the early stages of her infection. She took one GSE capsule three times a day. After only a few days, the infection cleared up. Karen is now a convert and grateful to be saving herself the antibiotic aftermath.

Chapter 13

MINIMIZE YOUR BEAUTY WILD CARDS

Beauty wild cards are the factors we can't always control. Wild cards such as the growing risks of standard healthcare, prescription-drug side effects, unresolved health and hormone issues, stress, and depression can jeopardize our precious vitality and our future in a wink. We can and must take steps to minimize them, if profound radiance is the goal.

step 1: learn about your own health issues

In today's awkward transitional period, at the dawn of the most major medical upheaval in history, we need to be armed with our own working knowledge of both our issues and our options so as not to fall victim to the current power struggle between the past and future of healthcare. Doing your own homework on your own health matters is a necessary part of self-preservation. Inform yourself on your issues and bring any proven therapies that could upgrade drugs without dangerous side effects to the attention of your doctor. If his or her mind is open, your doctor is a keeper; if he or she rejects your suggestions without explanation or exploration, find another doctor.

Regardless of what you've heard, some of the best information you can get is available on the Internet. There are also many cutting-edge books that will expand your perspective of your options as well. Look for them at health-food stores and at bookstores. See "Suggested Reading" in the Resources. Remember that you may need to inform your conventional doctor about these options, since most doctors are not given incentives to read studies on natural therapies and they can get into trouble for recommending solutions without FDA approval, no matter how much good science supports them. Doctors also have a limited area of specialty. Just as your neurologist may know little about your gynecological issues, there may be blind spots in your doctor's knowledge when it comes to natural or nutritional therapies.

step 2: don't risk your beauty with standard care

The most expensive, high-tech healthcare in the world has put the United States in about seventeenth place in life-expectancy, behind countries that spend up to 75 percent less on healthcare, according to the World Health Organization. Sixty-one percent of Americans are overweight or obese, and 125 million have one or more chronic diseases. This isn't a pretty picture.

Although most Americans believe that we have the best healthcare system in the world, the facts do not support this:

Risk of prescription drugs. According to the latest available figures from the *Journal of the American Medical Association*, properly prescribed and used prescription drugs cause over 106,000 deaths each year, making it the fourth leading cause of death (more than AIDS and gun fatalities combined). Iatrogenic—or conventional-treatment-caused—fatalities account for more than 225,000 deaths per year.

Drug recalls. More drugs have been recalled in the last fifteen years than in all of history.

Hospital facts. A 1999 Institute of Medicine report concluded that medical errors contribute to more than one million injuries and up to ninety-eight thousand deaths annually. A follow-up study published in the September 9, 2002, *Archives of Internal Medicine* noted that errors occurred in nearly one in five doses in a typical three-hundred-bed hospital, which translates to about two errors per patient daily.

Advertising. In 1997 the FDA granted drug companies the right to sell directly to consumers through television advertisements. Commercials have resulted in huge increases in prescription-drug use and an increased number of patients calling and visiting their doctor to get advertised drugs.

Get to the Bottom of Your Health Issues

The average doctor's appointment is down to 7½ minutes. It's no wonder we're so often discouraged from getting to the cause of our health complaints. I have annoyed many doctors by interrupting the often hasty process of assigning a drug to my condition by asking them to help me get to the cause of the problem. This is especially challenging under normal time constraints if they can't find an immediate and clear diagnosis. The easily recognizable diseases that can be categorized and to which drugs can readily be assigned usually develop long after subtle symptoms arise. This is when your conventional doctor may feel the most useful and can write a prescription for lifelong "control." So in effect, if you are patient and let low-grade complaints go their course with the help of over-the-counter symptom-mufflers, modern medicine will have a treatment once the disease reaches a full-blown state.

Favoring health-building, proven, natural approaches over symptom-blocking drugs that allow the original problem to progress is a crucial principle of self-preservation and pro-beauty living. Question any health practitioner who urges you at the first sign of trouble to forego the possibility of function-restoring health approaches in favor of far more costly, risky, short-sighted "fixes." Remember, medicine is a business, and your doctor is a businessman and a human being, just like the person who fixes your car—although your car might get more time! Aim higher for yourself, and find a doctor who serves your agenda.

Keep Your Doctor in Line with Your Objectives

You must operate on the health motive, even if your doctor is focused on your symptom. Lack of basic information is what put Fen-phen users at risk for permanent health problems in the 1990s.

There have always been doctors who are more than willing to help us hurt ourselves, but many draw the line when it comes to encouraging us to take clinically proven supplements or employ alternative healing methods to help ourselves live better lives while minimizing prescription-drug commitments. If you always opt first for the drug without considering non-drug therapies, you not only reward the million-dollar PR and sales force who educate your doctor and dominate his treatment repertoire but you also keep yourself in their sickness domain.

Second Opinions Are Crucial

If surgery or long-term prescription-drug therapy is recommended for your health issue, a second opinion from a complementary doctor or naturopathic physician who specializes in treating your condition can be an important measure in self-preservation and in ensuring the best perspective on your options.

Dr. David G. Edelson, founder of HealthBridge, a state-of-the-art New York–based integrative medical facility, stresses that second opinions shouldn't come from a practitioner who completely rejects drugs or surgery. Doctors must be able to recognize when a situation requires intervention, as was the case with one patient who risked kidney failure because his herbalist didn't realize his symptoms had reached a critical stage.

step 3: get a real checkup

Integrative or complementary physicians combine the diagnostic technology of conventional doctors with extensive nutritional and alternative perspectives and, where truly necessary, drugs or surgery. The truth is that conditions like mild depression, mild hypertension, and high cholesterol are often reversible without drugs. Even when drugs and surgery are used for other conditions, studies consistently show that they have better results when combined with nutritional and alternative therapies. If no crisis exists, you can spare yourself all kinds of misery and preserve your vitality by exploring nondrug solutions before problems get serious.

CHECKUP CHECKLIST

- Find a nutrition-oriented physician (see the Resources).
- Get copies of all blood work, X-ray results, and medical records.
- Keep a list of all drugs you're taking and their known side effects.
- Write down all symptoms and take them to your appointment.
- Get a full analysis of your blood, urine, hair (if possible), hormones, and bone density (after thirty-five), as well as a colon-cancer screening (particularly after fifty).
- Get screened if you suspect food or environmental allergies.
- Ask to have your homocysteine levels checked as well as your ratio of LDL (bad) to HDL (good) cholesterol levels.
- Bring any studies you have come across regarding safer alternatives proven to help your condition.

For organizations that can help you find a doctor who really listens to your complaints, who answers to science rather than pharmaceutical companies, and who is both amenable and knowledgeable with regard to nutritional talk, see the Resources.

Keep your own "wellness file" to help you keep track of your health history and take command over your healthcare objectives. Your wellness file should consist of your medical records, X rays, a list of the prescription drugs you're taking and their side effects, a list of your symptoms, even if they seem unrelated to your conditions, a list of allergies and food issues, the supplements you're taking, your lifestyle challenges, and key stress issues.

step 4: get a handle on your hormone issues and options

Hormone replacement therapy (HRT) should be an issue we can confidently work out with our doctors, but up until the fall of 2002 the odds were that your doctor was unlikely to know about plant-based or bio-identical hormones. In August 2002 the National Institute of Health's Women's Health Initiative study on HRT was halted after showing higher breast cancer, heart attack, and blood-clot risk in women taking the synthetic hormones for five years. Furthermore, few if any of the major health promises we'd been lured with have been delivered by synthetic HRT.

In the July 9, 2002, *New York Times* article on the study, Dr. Victoria Kusiak, the Vice President of Clinical Affairs and North American Medical Director at Wyeth, the largest maker of the hormone supplements, emphasized that there were "no other effective treatments for the symptoms of menopause." But GlaxoSmithKline simultaneously sent its sales force out with free samples and literature on Remifemin, its proprietary herbal preparation—*blends* of herbs can be patented, by the way—containing black cohosh, which was proven in placebo-controlled clinical trials in the '80s and '90s to offer equivalent—and in many regards, superior—effects to standard synthetic HRT in relieving hot flashes, psychological symptoms, and vaginal dryness. If the immediate jump in sales of the leading botanical menopause preparations were any indication, millions of eyes were suddenly opened to the possible benefits of natural plant estrogens and to herbal remedies in general.

The Soy Debate

You've probably heard about the benefits of soy and how the Japanese who eat a lot of it have fewer menopausal symptoms and fewer cases of breast cancer and heart disease. But you should be aware that there is some negative science out there amidst the positive science.

In the October 2002 edition of her newsletter, *The Lark Letter*, Dr. Susan Lark explained that the handful of negative studies on soy lose their significance in the face of hundreds of studies supporting the benefits of soy, including a July 2002 study published in *Cancer Epidemiology, Biomarkers, and Prevention*. The study found that women who ate soy-rich diets were 55 percent less likely to have abnormal breast-tissue growth than women who consumed the least soy.

On the other side of the fence, Harvard-trained Dr. Jonathan V. Wright, another highly respected complementary physician, wrote in his bulletin, *The Soy Myth Exposed*, that research points to processed soy powder's action in blocking certain important nutrients in one study. He also noted that certain chemicals in soy have been linked with increased incidence of an early form of breast malignancy and metastasis. The objective truth here is that there are still hundreds of studies showing the benefits of soy and only a handful of negative ones. (To order these articles or subscribe to either of these doctors' informative newsletters, see the Resources.)

Many women with mild hormonal imbalances and PMS can get substantial relief by making lifestyle upgrades and taking supportive supplements such as black cohosh, dong quai, and chaste tree berry. But there is more substantial relief for those who've been thrown off-balance by their hormonal issues thanks to standardized, plant-based HRT, or bio-identical HRT, which have not shown any of the immediate or long-term risks inherent to synthetic HRT.

Hormones are different from other supplements, though. You need to be monitored and supervised by a doctor, since it's too easy to get off-balance. And before you make any decisions, I advise you to read a good book on the subject, such as one by Dr. Christiane Northrup or Dr. John Lee (see the Resources). For the best results, find a doctor, gynecologist, or naturopath who is knowledgeable in the use of bio-identical estrogen and natural progesterone therapies and who works with a compounding pharmacist to formulate individualized therapies for each woman.

Estrogen Dominance: Bad for Your Health, Not to Mention Your Hips

You already know what insulin and stress hormones can do to your shape, but did you know that excess estrogen can also cause the body to hoard fat? According to Dr. Lark, estrogen dominance can become a problem with age that often begins in your thirties. In addition to heavy and irregular menstrual periods and other gynecological issues, estrogen promotes the deposition of fat typical to the female configuration—in the hip area—and fluid retention within the tissues, she says. To help correct estrogen dominance nutritionally she recommends ground flaxseed and other fibers that bind with estrogen and fat and promote their elimination from the body. Fish and fish-oil supplements, vitamin B6, vitex, and most importantly, a good multivitamin and mineral regimen can help maintain a healthy estrogen balance. The liver plays a big part in detoxifying estrogen, so taking detoxifying measures, such as reducing alcohol consumption, can help, says Lark. Natural progesterone therapy can also balance estrogen levels. A good complementary physician or naturopathic doctor can guide you on how to maintain this balance.

CAFFEINE RAISES ESTROGEN

Dr. Lark points out that caffeine from all sources has been linked with higher estrogen. A 2001 study published in *Fertility and Sterility* showed that women who drank four to five cups per day produced nearly 70 percent more estrogen than those who consumed less than one cup. This study is reinforced by two earlier studies published in the *International Journal of Cancer* that linked caffeine with PMS and increased ovarian cancer risk in premenopausal women.

Check Your Thyroid

Thyroid problems are major beauty and quality-of-life issues that often go undetected. If you're cold all the time, can't lose weight, are tired, or have droopy lids, sparse eyebrows, brittle hair, or dry skin, get your thyroid hormone levels checked. But realize that even if your doctor's test comes back normal, conventional thyroid hormone tests are notorious for missing real thyroid issues since blood levels of the hormone do not reflect thyroid function. The Broda O. Barnes, M.D., Foundation, a nonprofit organization considered to be the premiere educational organization on thyroid issues (see the Resources for contact information), established the Barnes Basal Body Temperature self-test that you can do at home. It is considered the most reliable indicator of thyroid function by complementary and alternative doctors (see sidebar for the test).

If your temperature reading is in the below-normal range, doctors will often prescribe a trial prescription of synthetic thyroid hormone, though a natural dessicated bovine thyroid called Armour Thyroid may have advantages due to a broader spectrum of hormones, according to a letter by Dr. Alan Gaby to the *Journal of the American Medical Association*. A 1999 study published in *The New England Journal of Medicine* showed that patients had greater improvements in mood when they were treated with Armour Thyroid as opposed to Synthroid.

THE BARNES BASAL BODY TEMPERATURE SELF-TEST

Basal temperatures are taken first thing in the morning before you get out of bed and when your body is completely at rest. Menstruating women must take this test on the second, third, and fourth days of their periods only. Non-menstruating women, women who have had hysterectomies, and men can take their temperature at any time.

The night before you take the test, do not drink any alcohol. Shake a glass mercury thermometer down and leave it by your bed. In the morning, before getting out of bed and with as little movement as possible, place the thermometer under your arm and leave it there for ten minutes.

The normal temperature range is 97.8–98.2. A lower temperature means you might be a candidate for thyroid hormone therapy. If your thyroid function is borderline-sluggish, a nutrition-oriented doctor may recommend supplements such as kelp and L-tyrosine to stimulate thyroid function.

step 5: strategize creatively against stress, sleep, and mood issues

Another hormone that wreaks havoc is cortisol. Stress and a lack of deep sleep can lead to elevated levels of cortisol, which can in turn cause a cascade of immune and inflammatory issues, like skin eruptions, tissue and muscle breakdown, fat accumulation and edema, bone loss, and thyroid imbalances. In his book *Caffeine Blues*, Stephen Cherniske, M.S., notes that overworked women may have higher than normal cortisone levels. As mentioned in chapter 5, caffeine can contribute to these issues, since it causes the release of stress hormones and raises cortisol. High levels of cortisol can destroy our bones. Cherniske refers to a study by Phillip Gold, a researcher at the National Institutes of Mental Health in Bethesda, Maryland, that compared bone mineral density in women with both normal and elevated cortisol and found those with elevated stress hormones had the bone density similar to that of seventy-year-olds.

In one double-blind, placebo-controlled study published in the *International Journal of Sports Medicine*, plant sterolins were found to have a buffering effect on many stress-induced factors, including cortisol levels and inflammation in marathon runners. (See the Resources for plant sterolins.) The supplement Relora also looks very promising as a means to control cortisol, but more research needs to be done to confirm preliminary findings. You can be updated on such developments through my educational Web site, *www.informedbeauty.com*, and through other organizations, newsletters, and on-line sources listed in the Resources.

Last, but certainly not least, exercise, particularly in meditative forms, such as yoga and t'ai chi, can effectively reduce stress and cortisol levels while improving your overall health. Try yoga by joining a class or purchasing a good video or book. If you are already an avid fitness buff, keep

EXERCISE: THE ULTIMATE ANTIDEPRESSANT

A team of Duke University Medical Center researchers demonstrated in late 1999 that thirty minutes either riding a stationary bike, walking, or jogging three times a week was just as effective after sixteen weeks as Zoloft in treating major depression in the middle-aged and elderly.

in mind that overexercise, both chronically or at one time, can cause cortisol to kick in and become a problem. If you're an all-or-nothing type or a weekend warrior, understand the importance of balance here.

Relieve Your Stress Creatively

- Express yourself—speak up!
- Pursue your passion.
- If you feel trapped, set new boundaries.
- Choose activities the encourage you to tune in to yourself, not tune out.
- Keep a journal.
- Get/spend time with a pet.
- Read books that address your emotional issues.
- Spend time with people who expect great things of you.
- Be active in a way you enjoy.
- Support yourself nutritionally with stress adaptogens like ginseng and plant sterolins.

Take Your Beauty Sleep Seriously

Getting your beauty sleep goes way beyond the avoidance of under-eye circles. It can greatly affect your health and even your weight. It is during "deep-wave" sleep that hormone activities—like the release of human growth hormone (hGH) and regulation of cortisol—really kick in, protecting us from inflammation, the cumulative aging effects of stress, and other cortisol-related effects such as weight gain in the belly and immune problems. HGH is the body's fountain of youth, keeping skin thick and supple and the body lean and muscular. It also helps keep every other system in the body energized and in working order.

- Getting some sun early in the day and using a sleep mask at night will help your body produce more melatonin, which helps you sleep.

- Nose strips, anti-snore sprays, and pillows that support the neck can reduce or stop snoring, which interferes with deep sleep.
- Upgrade coffee or alcohol to herbal nightcaps for deeper sleep.
- Herbs and supplements such as valerian and 5Htp have proven relaxing effects.
- Hypo-allergenic and dust-mite-proof bedding can vastly improve your mornings and your under-eye circles, if you deal with allergies (see the Resources).

Detoxify Your Emotions

Emotional issues affect us all, right down to our cells. Detoxifying your emotions is an ongoing part of the shedding process. In your dawn-to-dusk self-inventory, you identified the daily patterns and triggers that shape your mood curve. Paying close attention to your emotions will help you understand how they affect your life and body.

I still work on tons of emotional issues even though my eating disorder is history. I've had my own breakthroughs with the help of solitude, creative pursuits, journal writing, and hours in bookstores. Even if you get counseling, you still have to do positive activities on your own. Resonating book passages, meditating, giving yourself emotional space, finding a new creative pursuit, and reading an old journal entry can all neutralize and diffuse negative self-talk and emotional triggers that lead to bingeing and other forms of self-sabotage.

If you suspect you're depressed, it is important to seek professional help. Talk with someone and keep them apprised of how you're doing, no matter what degree of depression you're feeling. Depression, like any illness, happens for a reason. We should listen to it and use it as it begins to set in. There are many nutritional supplements and herbal remedies that have been shown by solid research to lift mild to moderate depression without the serious side effects associated with prescription antidepressants.

Read about them in a number of books and educational channels listed in the Resources.

Solitude and boundaries are also important. They are often elusive if you have kids or live with people who don't respect your emotional boundaries. You have to make a concerted effort to draw the lines. If your life doesn't allow for some solitude and self-determined activities, you must take steps to secure set boundaries that cannot be broken. And you must set emotional boundaries between you and anyone close to you who might be interfering with your ability to do what's best for yourself.

Build Yourself Up with the Process of Shedding

The process of shedding is powerful enough to revese the downward cycle of self-sabotage and lift you up, one act at a time. Your subconscious picks up on each positive act and becomes increasingly responsive to the special treatment you are giving yourself. As you feel the burdens that once endangered your beauty melt away with each new choice, you will also feel your spirit lift and an increased sense of self-respect.

Chapter 14

MAKE LIFE
AN AUTHENTIC
BEAUTY RITUAL

Throughout the course of this book I've applied the three tools—
the magic motivation of health, complete information,
and access to the best resources—to each area of our
dawn-to-dusk lives. With these powerful new tools and
the Resources in the final section of this book, you now
have everything you need to become your own passionate connoisseur.

As you finish reading this book, return to your dawn-
to-dusk self-inventory and choose your first cycle of
strategic, pro-beauty upgrades. As each cycle of shedding and upgrades becomes second nature and propels
itself into the next, you'll release more burdens and side-
step countless new challenges. You'll soon become adept
at tapping the transformative power that lies dormant
in every choice until no choice remains mundane in your
evolving recipe for self-creation. You'll gain an exhilarat-
ing new sense of freedom and awareness that will

empower and uplift you in unimagined ways, and you'll continually set your own criteria for what goes on in your body and how you live. As you cultivate yourself with growing clarity and the ever-expanding options that enable you to have it all, your concept of the good life, the nature of your beauty splurges, your spirit, and the person staring back at you from your mirror will never be the same. And here's the most amazing part: Once your tastes, your concept of decadence, and your desires have evolved to become one and the same with your body's innate desires, you are home free. You will have achieved a state I affectionately call "beauty nirvana," an effortless, joyful state that lifts you in an upward spiral toward nature's intention: an ageless beauty that is never static.

shedding frees us up for more purposeful pursuits

The beautiful thing about the process of shedding is that it frees up so much energy that was once tied up in the old merry-go-round. Each of us has gifts we've either cultivated or neglected. Now is the time to focus your newfound energy into that greater purpose. Vitality is the point where our physical manifestation connects with our inner spirit, and when all is said and done, what comes from that spirit is what really counts. Vitality and radiance are simply joyful mediums for the expression of our truest gifts from the heart.

cultivate your intrinsic beauty

When we are disconnected with our unique essence, there is a hole in our foundation for self-creation. Discounting the inner wisdom we are born with is like asking the painter Gaugin, "Which artists have influenced you?" and then shaming him for daring to say his work came from his own soul. We have so much inside that we've been shamed out of tapping into it and expressing it by parents, siblings, co-workers, spouses, and others whose approval we seek or who are threatened by the part of us they can't understand or control. I have worked with women whose gurus, hairstyles, designer clothes, facialists, bikini waxers, and pilates instructors are the same as their mother's or their friends'. These women fear they might fall out of favor if they were to go in their own direction or make some of those choices privately. A different situation has been described by many of my Web site readers who have shared their battles with husbands who unwittingly contribute to their struggles with food by interfering with their attempts to break their own patterns or establish needed boundaries. It takes vigilance to establish and defend our own boundaries. By giving others the space and unconditional support that fosters and encourages their own self-creation, you set the stage for granting yourself that same nonjudgmental room to explore, fail, and grow as you embark on the unbeaten path to your own truest purpose.

Vitality is the point where our physical manifestation connects with our inner spirit.

Perhaps the real key to developing our independent spirit is not in finding the time or the right group with which to pursue a spiritual path but to find ways to avoid having our own innate spirit trampled or imposed upon. We need to give our own inner wisdom its platform within our hearts. Evolve your self through self-knowledge and truth and what they lead you to. Draw on the wisdom of others, but don't accept that your own unique collection of beliefs and instincts are inferior in any way to any other belief systems.

using our most beautiful gifts

What's even more important than the gifts we possess is how we channel and use them. There are so many passionate and bright people whose gifts fail to manifest their much-needed good to the world. This quiz was forwarded to me by e-mail (author unknown). It is a beautiful testament to the nature of our truest gifts:

1. Name the five wealthiest people in the world.
2. Name the last five Heisman Trophy winners.
3. Name the last five winners of the Miss America contest.
4. Name ten people who have won the Nobel or Pulitzer Prize.
5. Name the last half-dozen Academy Award winners for Best Actor and Best Actress.
6. Name the last decade's World Series winners.

How did you do?

The point is that none of us remembers yesterday's headliners. They're the best in their fields, but the applause dies, awards tarnish, achievements are forgotten, and accolades and certificates are buried with their owners.

Now here's another quiz. See how you do on this one:

1. List a few teachers who aided your journey through school.
2. Name three friends who helped you through a difficult time.
3. Name five people who taught you something worthwhile.
4. Think of a few people who make you feel appreciated and special.
5. Think of five people you enjoy spending time with.
6. Name a half-dozen heroes whose stories have inspired you.

Easier? The lesson: The people who make a difference in your life aren't the ones with the most credentials, the most money, or the most awards. They're the ones who care.

let your beauty ripple outward

Another potential gift each of us can give to the world is a passion for the stories and the values behind the products we buy. My own passionate pursuit of high-quality products and meaningful services and support for pro-beauty living has led me to some of the most amazing and passionate people I've ever encountered. One couple who knew nothing about organic farming developed one of the most profitable organic-produce companies in the world out of a strong desire to do something for the environment and for people. A maker of some of the purest body-care products I've found healed herself of non-Hodgkin's lymphoma by detoxifying her life and using homegrown herbs in her microbatch body delicacies. The creator of one of the most cutting-edge supplement lines transformed himself from diseased and emaciated to healthy and robust. These are people and companies after my own heart. We share a creative spirit that has come out of transforming our own lives and the need to share what we have learned and created with others. There are no spokespeople or number-crunchers fronting or vouching for or compromising the quality of these products. These products and companies are as rare, real, and precious as the most beautiful endangered butterfly. If we want the hope of a more beautiful future, we have to seek out companies that reflect what we want to see more of in the world. Capture this beauty and make these companies a part of your life. Many of them are listed in the Resources.

THE REAL BEAUTY SPLURGES

- Pure, live food
- Pure water
- Pure air
- Pure, potent, and proven personal-care products
- High-quality supplements
- High-quality healthcare

Discover even more of them at your natural-product, specialty, and vitamin stores and on-line.

guard your beauty with your life

As connoisseurs and cultivators of our beauty and our lives, we need uninterrupted access to true sustenance and untainted raw materials. If we want continued access to food that still has nutrients and life force in it; water that doesn't harm us more than it helps us; clean, quality seafood; pure body-care products; quality supplements; and innovative, accountable healthcare, we need to express these demands through our choices and recognize their true value by being willing to pay for it. We mustn't take these precious needs for granted. Beauty has no real future without them.

stay aware, stay beautiful

It has never been more important for each of us to understand the issues that occasionally threaten the future of our beauty and quality of life. Fortunately it has never been easier to get hooked in to the resources that can elevate our quality of life and to the complete, unfiltered, and unpackaged information we need to stay ahead of the game and steer clear of beauty wild cards.

the other pro-beauty choice issues

Since 1989, industries have contributed more than $68 million to political candidates who support laws that allow them to release untold chemicals into the environment. Other laws sweeping through Europe threaten our future freedom to improve our health and quality of life with supplements. And the agricultural biotechnology seen by many scientists as an uncontrollable threat to the world's food supply is running neck and neck with the emerging hope of sustainable agriculture and the unstoppable passion of consumers.

On top of all of this lies the inarguable fact that globalization gives corporations unprecedented protection from accountability to our health, our environment, and our quality of life. Fortunately, this disturbing reality is still exquisitely vulnerable to the power of your choice. More than fifty million people in this country are actively seeking deeper meaning in their choices, purchases, and lives, and this passion is felt and quantified with fascination by economists and market analysts. We are in an age of great upheaval. The medical guard is changing, and many current practices will soon be relegated to the archives of a medical Dark Age. Agriculture is changing. Environmental frivolity is becoming intolerable, even to the mainstream. Fat-free is over. Consumers' blind faith is over. For the uninformed, life will continue to get worse before it gets better, but for the informed, it can be better than ever right now.

stand up for your beauty and your quality of life

Though it may seem daunting to be up against polluters and soulless corporations that don't want consumers to be informed, consumers have begun to make a huge difference with their dollars and with their computers. Perhaps the most exciting contribution that computers have made to society is their ability to connect and mobilize huge numbers of people in support of important issues. One of the most encouraging examples of this new kind of grass-roots power was demonstrated in the late 1990s, when efforts by over fifty organizations informed and mobilized an unprecedented 275,603 Americans to e-mail comments and successfully defeat the USDA's attempt to degrade the definition of organic-food standards to include GMO foods and other potential health hazards. Several important organizations representing the crucial issues that can make or break our quality of life have made the act of raising our voices as easy as a couple of mouse clicks. You can certainly make a difference without a computer as well. See the Resources for a list of organizations that will inform and inspire you to make a difference.

save your own beauty and you help save the world

It used to be nearly impossible or at least inconvenient to reconcile your desire for high-end results and appeal with your desire to do no harm to yourself or the planet in the process. But for the first time in history, you no longer need to compromise any of those desires. It is now easy, pleasant, and more rewarding than ever to live in harmony with the values so many of us have suppressed within ourselves for far too long. Corporations that make mediocre, harmful, and polluting products are now at your mercy like never before. Start with your choices on a personal level to turn the tide. Let your own beauty ripple outward and you can begin to save the world.

take your tools along for the journey

No one can or should tell you how to proceed from here. Part of the power of shedding is the joyful spirit of discovery and creativity that feeds your own unique process. All you need to take with you from here are your new tools. Keep them honed and by your side and they will surely take you where you want to go. Shedding is forever. Enjoy the process.

the living beauty resource guide

The following is a special collection of rare and one-of-a-kind products, services, and support that lets you expand your own standard for the good life wherever you live. Most of the products mentioned throughout the previous chapters, as well as many of the products here, are available from natural-foods stores and other retailers of natural products. Where noted, you can also call or visit the company's Web site. Availability may change or products may be discontinued, but rest assured that better products are being created every day for the new kind of consumer this guide is designed to please. Because new products are introduced all the time, I encourage you to visit my Web site, *www.informedbeauty.com*, for new and additional product information.

Finally, I've also included a listing of some of the most reliable resources for staying on top of new science and quality-of-life issues in your areas of interest. Welcome to a world where science and companies serve *you*, where substance counts and so does the impact of your choice. Everyone should live this well!

foods and beverages

Almond Butter by Maranatha, Woodstock Farms, and other brands

The ultimate to your body is organic, *raw* almond butter; most kinds are roasted.

Amy's Soy Macaroni and Cheese

Tastes like the real thing and is more real than most other frozen versions. Find it in the health-food freezer section.

Bearitos Organic Microwave Popcorn

Non-hydrogenated, unlike nearly all the other microwaveable popcorn. Melt real organic butter over this and sneak it into the movies!

Bonterra Organic Wines

This is one of several fine, organically produced wines. It has little or no preservatives, including sulfites, such as are present in other organic wines. For some, this could mean a way to enjoy wine without the headaches and under-eye circles. Ask your liquor store to order it.

Breads

Alvarado Street Bakery breads, bagels, and buns

No white bread can come close to the taste of these sprouted breads, buns, and bagels. (The onion/poppy-seed bagel is the best store-bought bagel there is.) The breads make fantastic avocado sandwiches, bread pudding, and French toast. Don't buy these breads if you're addicted to carbs, or at least consider taking a phaseolamin-based supplement before eating them.

La Tortilla Factory Low Carb Tortillas

www.latortillafactory.com

You don't have to give up tortillas or taste with these. I love the green onion flavor and use these in breakfast burritos, quesadillas, wraps, and pizzas. Unlike some low-carb foods, they contain no unhealthy ingredients or trans-fats.

Manna Bread

This is a one-of-a-kind "bread" that is flourless, moist, sprouted, and so alive and perishable that it must be stored in the freezer and kept refrigerated once opened. I take one dense slice and add a generous dollop of almond butter, which lowers its glycemic index. Find it in the freezer at your health-food store.

Chocolate, Gourmet Dark

Green and Black's

www.greenandblacks.com

Green and Black's Maya Gold, with spicy orange and vanilla bean extracts, is made from cocoa beans farmed by indigenous Mayans in Belize. The hazelnut and currant is also amazing. Though still dark, these are slightly sweeter than Taste Therapy.

Taste Therapy Chocolate for the Soul
by Endangered Species Chocolate Company

541-535-2170 • *www.chocolatebar.com*

This very dark bar knocked me off my feet. Neroli, from orange blossoms, has unique qualities that benefit the skin, but now I have experienced how it can benefit the soul. The sugar content is 8 grams (less than a glass of milk), and the organic cocoa solids are at a body-decadent 70 percent.

Chocolate, Low-Carb

Atkins Endulge Bars

800-6-ATKINS • *www.atkinscenter.com*

Carbolite Chocolate

www.carbolitedirect.com

Keto Nuts Macadamia (chocolate covered)

800-542-3230 • *www.lifeservices.com*

Pure De-Lite

888-569-2272 • *www.lowcarbliving.com*

Find these maltitol or Splenda (Sucralose)–sweetened treats at vitamin and health-food stores. Pure De-Lite's chocolate is Belgian. Atkins's Crunch is a dead ringer for Nestle's Crunch.

Cracker Flax

This one-of-a-kind, low-glycemic cracker will scratch your munchie itch without the carb consequences. Dip the onion-tomato flavor in your favorite hummus, or dip the apple-raisin in yogurt or almond butter for excellent munching.

Designer Protein by Next Proteins

This is one of several companies that makes the superior, highly digestible and utilized ion-exchange form of whey protein. Designer Protein comes in a natural flavor, without Acesulfame K or other artificial sweeteners and flavors. This is a versatile way to add high-quality, super-absorbable protein to just about anything from cereal to yogurt to shakes. It's 97 percent lactose-free.

Earthbound Farm washed organic salad greens

Look for these convenient organic lettuces, already washed and ready to eat, in refrigerated health-food produce sections. Add walnuts, avocado or other good protein, olive, grapeseed, or walnut oil to make a meal. Slivers of pear and red onion, a pinch of basil, and freshly ground pepper make it heaven.

Eden Organic Black Soybeans

Perhaps the healthiest and most versatile canned food, soybeans are the lowest-carb legume. They stand in perfectly for high-carb black beans and conveniently add high-quality, tasty protein to soups, salads, and whole-grain pilafs.

Fish, Gourmet and Sustainable

EcoFish

877-214-FISH • *www.ecofish.com*

EcoFish can deliver wild Alaskan salmon and other premium sustainable fish to you from anywhere in the country. If you want better fish and want to insure its availability in the future, start here. Buying the right kind of fish is not only win-win; it's crucial.

Dave's Gourmet Albacore

888-454-8862 • *www.davesalbacore.com.*

This premium and eco-friendly canned fish may just be the best available, and you can feel good about eating it. Water-packed albacore tuna is rich in omega-3s.

Meat and Poultry, Free-Range

Coleman Beef

www.colemannatural.com

Top-quality, certified organic beef that is widely available.

Green Circle Organics

www.greencircle.com

Top-grade, certified organic black Angus that is grass-fed and then grain-"finished" for slight marbling. Available at Whole Foods and other fine stores.

Eberly Poultry

www.eberlypoultry.com

Shelton's Free Range Turkey Italian Sausage

Find these in the natural-foods-store freezer section. Serve the sausage with low-carb spaghetti for a new and improved classic dish.

Juices

R. K. Knudson and *Lakewood* unsweetened cranberry and pomegranate juices. The former is proven effective against bladder infections. The latter fights heart disease.

Kefir (Unsweetened)

Kefir is basically drinkable yogurt, which is great for digestion, health, and the skin. Few people who are intolerant of milk have trouble digesting naturally fermented yogurt or kefir because the live active bacteria cultures actually digest most of the lactose. Try it in smoothies with Designer Protein, fruit, and healthy sweetener.

Low-Carb Munchies

These sources carry low-carb snacks, bake mixes, pastas, breads, chips, cereals, cheesecakes, ice-cream mixes, and more.

Atkins Direct

800-6-ATKINS • *www.atkinscenter.com*

Low Carb Creations

800-896-3405 • *www.getlowcarbcreations.com*

Keto Foods

800-542-3230 • *www.ketofoods.com*

Kat James's Low-Carb Connoisseur's Samplers

Order from *www.informedbeauty.com*

Some low-carb stuff tastes good, some doesn't. I have selected some of the best-tasting items that will pass muster with finicky family members. Three different samplers vary in price and products but include some or all of the following low-carb or sugar-free items: Lo Han Sweet pasta (don't overcook it!), apple-and-cinnamon hot cereal, banana-walnut pancake mix, Belgian chocolate bars, the best-tasting chips, onion and garlic bagels, soft tortillas, and more.

Lo Han Sweet™ Powder Sweetness Enhancer by Jarrow Formulas

Available through *www.webvitamins.com* and other natural-products retailers
A combination of naturally sweet xylitol and a compound from the Lo Han fruit from southern China. It's more than two hundred times sweeter than sugar yet does not cause blood-sugar swings. Xylitol lends a cool, sweet taste and is actually good for the teeth and body.

Oils and Vinegars

Jean-Georges California Grapeseed Oil

A product from four-star chef Jean-Georges Vongerichten. Known for its light taste, ability to withstand high cooking temperatures, and health properties, grapeseed oil also raises good and lowers bad cholesterol.

Meyer Lemon by Napa Valley Harvest

707-252-WINE • *www.winecountrykitchens.com*
A wonderful, versatile lemon-spiked grapeseed oil spritzer that puts salads, vegetables, and stir-fries over the top. Finish with roasted sesame and chili oils if you want a killer Asian stir-fry!

Organic Balsamic Vinegar by Monari Federzoni

Always use any vinegar with some oil to slow its sugar (glycemic) impact.

Organic olive oil and balsamic vinegar (sulfite-free) companion cruets by Gaeta Imports • *www.gaetaimports.com*

These cruets make an elegant gift.

Spectrum Naturals

These cold-pressed organic oils—grapeseed, sesame, flax, canola, and coconut—are pure and hexane- and trans-fat-free. Coconut is great for cooking.

Old Savanahh Gingerbread Mix

This 100 percent whole-wheat, non-hydrogenated mix is good and spicy. I made a gingerbread house out of it once. Carb addicts, take precautions!

Organic Produce Delivered to Your Door

Diamond Organics

888-ORGANIC • *www.diamondorganics.com*

Organic produce delivered to most areas of the United States overnight.

Urban Organic

718-499-4321 • *www.urbanorganic.net*

Delivers to the East-coast tri-state area

Local Harvest

www.localharvest.org

Can help you locate organic farmers near you, wherever you live.

Organic Gourmet sauces, mixes, and spices

800-400-7772 • *www.organic-gourmet.com*

Old-fashioned sauce and gravy mixes, mushroom and miso stocks, vegetable bouillon cubes without additives like MSG and hydrolyzed vegetable oil. They also carry organic peppercorns and other spice-rack staples.

Pastas, Low-Carb and Whole-Grain

Keto Low-carb Spaghetti

800-542-3230 • *www.lifeservices.com*

At this writing, this is the only good-tasting, truly low-carb pasta choice.

Eddie's Organic Soy Pasta
Edenfoods Brown Rice, Soba, and Buckwheat Pastas

These pastas are higher-carb than Keto brand though still far healthier than white-pasta choices. New healthier pastas are being produced every day, so keep your eyes open.

Pumpkin Seed Oil

North American Herb and Spice

800-243-5242

Flora

800-446-2110 • *www.florahealth.com*

This oil is so therapeutic that it is sometimes taken as a supplement, but the taste is unbelievable and will make any risotto, salad, or appetizer amazing. It's also a gift any gourmand would appreciate.

Pumpkorn

A great spicy pumpkinseed snack to eat on the run or at the movies. Keep it in your purse as a munchie to keep your energy level stable when you can't eat a real meal. Also great sprinkled on salads.

SlimSweet by TriMedica

www.trimedica.com

The only all-natural sweetener approved by the Glycemic Research Institute for use by most diabetics. A zero-calorie, naturally low-glycemic form of fructose from kiwi, clinically shown not to stimulate oversecretion of insulin. It's good as a sugar substitute, even in cooking, and ten times sweeter than ordinary fructose.

Sloppy Joe Mix by Simply Organic

I almost cried when I found this no-MSG, non-hydrolyzed mix for my famous free-range turkey sloppy joes! Do 'em up your way, but use sprouted or low-carb buns.

SoooLite! by NuNaturals

800-753-HERB • www.nunaturals.com

I love this zero-carb stevia product because it tastes the most like sugar. To achieve this, they naturally selected less bitter stevia plants for a non-GMO hybrid with no aftertaste.

Tamarind Tree Heat and Serve Indian Entrees

www.tamtree.com

The only heat-and-serve entrees with brown rice I have found! Navratan Korma is fresh vegetables, unsulphured raisins, pistachios, and almonds in a marinade of light cream and cashew paste. Exceptional convenience food.

Teas and Herbal Infusions

Celadon

510-524-1696 • *www.celadontea.com*

A wide range of fresh, fine teas, including the buttery Taiwanese Oolongs, such as their Tung Ting tea. Lychee fruit and Rose Red (black tea scented with rose) are other popular teas that don't need sugar.

In Pursuit of Tea

718-302-0780 • *www.truetea.com*

A wide variety, including Yinzhen Silver Needle white tea, the finest white tea available. With its downy, silvery hairs, it may even have health effects more powerful than green. Lowest in caffeine. Beautiful array of pots and accessories.

SpecialTeas

888-365-6983 • *www.specialteas.com*

Many rare teas and innovative blends, including Osmanthus green (green tea rolled with osmanthus blossoms), a fruity, peachy blend that will please former sugary fruit-tea addicts. Earl Grey rooibus is another novelty, and even a rooibus with bourbon-vanilla pieces. Try Berry Lapacho with black currant peaches (lapacho is a traditional health tonic that tastes like anything but).

Tisana traditional "liquid herbal dietary supplements"

Imported by Scarangello Company Inc.

800-871-4741 ext. 00 • *www.healthytea.biz*

Produced by Italy's leading herbal authority, Costanza Giunti. Extremely potent and used for hundreds of years in Europe, these results-driven drinkable herbs (thicker than tea) grown from mineral-rich, volcanic soil in Italy support various body systems and are featured at the finest tearooms and medi-spas here and abroad. Most decrease bloating, detoxify the liver, stimulate the lymphatic system, and have effects on the skin and even cellulite. Beauty elixirs at their best.

Hampstead premium biodynamic teas

www.affinityfoods.com

The first certified biodynamic (better than organic) single estate tea in the world. Harvested from the Makaibari estate in Darjeeling, India and certified by the Fair Trade Foundation. Connoisseurs will relish their First Flush Tea—the rare, tender pickings from the first leaves in spring.

Teeccino Herbal Coffee

800-498-3434 • *www.teeccino.com*

This is the best coffee upgrade I've found. It provides the taste, sensory experience, and brewing ritual of coffee. Find it in the coffee or tea section at health-food stores, or order direct.

Uncle Sam Cereal by U.S. Mills

Available at conventional and natural-food stores. This is a one-of-a-kind, low-glycemic, whole-wheat and flaxseed cereal that also happens to taste great and have amazing immediate effects on digestion as well as the countless skin and body benefits of flaxseed. If you're avoiding carbs, sprinkle over yogurt.

supplements

Most supplements discussed in this book are available in vitamin stores. The following is a list of stand-outs. See pages 304–5 for some great mail-order sources for supplements.

The development of transdermal products, sprays, and other forms of supplementation is happening too quickly to keep up with in any book. For updates on the new, scientifically proven transdermal patches and creams—and even clothing!—that deliver a growing variety of therapeutic substances (and even a proven fat emulsifier) directly into the body, visit my Web site at *www.informedbeauty.com.*

Please note that the listings and information below are not intended to diagnose or treat disease. Always enlist your doctor's supervision when addressing health complaints or illness with supplements or any other information in this book.

Advanced High-Potency Full-Spectrum Supplement Regimens

The regimens below contain therapeutic potencies and the most comprehensive spectrums of vitamins, minerals, superfoods, EFAs, and phytonutrients available. Each formula varies, so I advise you to look into specific nutrients that may serve you best.

Forward Plus Daily Regimen, created by Dr. Julian Whitaker
800-722-8008 • *www.drwhitaker.com*

Daily Advantage, created by Dr. David G. Williams
800-888-1415 • *www.drdavidwilliams.com*

Life Extension Mix from Life Extension Foundation
800-544-4440 • *www.lef.org*

Whole Food–Based Formulas by MegaFood, Garden of Life,
and New Chapter
www.megafood.com • *www.gardenoflifeusa.com* • *www.new-chapter.com*
MegaFood features Foodstate™ nutrients, which have been found to be more effective at inhibiting glycation than their isolated counterparts.[1] *Garden of Life* and *New Chapter* create state-of-the-art, fermented multivitamin, mineral, and herbal formulas with whole-food concentrates, enzymes, and ionic minerals that are far more available to the cells than those of most other vitamins,

Green Powders, Drinks, and Food Supplements

Green substances like wheat and barley grass, spirulina, and chlorella offer what it is lacking in the average American diet: body-detoxifying chlorophyll, enzymes, and important plant sources of vitamin B12, phytonutrients, enzymes, and amino acids. I've seen and experienced remarkable changes in energy, skin clarity, joint function, and appetite from taking them.

E3Live Wildgrown Superfood by Vision, Inc.
888-800-7070 (East Coast) or 888-233-1441 (West Coast) • *www.e3live.com*
This green food for connoisseurs (also popular with Olympic athletes) is the only blue-green algae product frozen fresh and delivered in its vital state. This is serious, expensive stuff. Users report amazing skin and health changes.

Perfect Food by Garden of Life
Contains more superfoods, antioxidant complexes, and organic green foods per serving than any other green powder.

Sun Chlorella Broken Cell Wall Chlorella by Sun Wellness, Inc.
Chlorella packs the highest concentration and delivery of chlorophyll and nucleic acids and has been shown to remove heavy metals from the body and shield cells from free-radical damage. Sun Chlorella features the broken cell wall for best absorption.

One-of-a-Kind Supplements

7-Keto™ Naturalean by Enzymatic Therapy

Naturalean by Enzymatic Therapy contains thyroid-supportive nutrients as well as 7-Keto™ DHEA, which is considered the safest form of DHEA. Published studies showed profound weight loss in those taking this supplement when compared to a placebo. DHEA supplements also alleviate depression while increasing libido and well-being. Take only under your doctor's supervision.

AdvaCal advanced calcium supplement by Lane Labs

Order from CompassioNet • 800-510-2010

This is the only calcium supplement proven at this writing to increase bone density.

Breast Health by Schiff

Contains detoxifying D-Glucarate and green tea, shown to offer some protection against breast cancer.

Carb Cutter, Carbo Tame, Carb Phaser, Cblock, and other phaseolamin-based supplements

Carb Cutter and Carb Phaser are available through vitamin retailers. CBlock can be ordered through Luminescence at 800-364-6637. These are key tools for the recovering carb addict. They block the enzyme that digests and converts carbs to fat, so they are largely passed through the body. Unlike fat blockers, they don't block important nutrients. Take half an hour before meals.

Carnosine and Chronoforte from Life Extension Foundation

800-544-4440 • www.lef.org.

Carnosine is the glycation-inhibiting supplement that may slow the aging process of glycation. Chronoforte is a serious antiaging combo of free radical–fighting acetyl L-Carnitine, antioxidant-recycling alpha-lipoic acid, glycation-fighting carnosine, cancer-preventing selenium, and inflammation-fighting nettle.

Daily Balance female support supplements, created by Dr. Susan Lark

888-314-5275 • www.drlark.com

Dr. Lark's PMS, Hot Flash, and Menorragia (heavy menstruation) supplements are cutting edge. Progest E, a natural progesterone in a spray, is also available.

FTF • *www.shopcyberworld.com*

FTF (Fight the Fat) is the only form of liquid chitosan (a shellfish substance that absorbs fat) which doesn't cause digestive funkiness and works immediately. Virtually tasteless and colorless. Avoid it if you're allergic to shellfish. Note that chitosan absorbs healthy fat, so limit use to large fatty meals, and don't take it when eating healthy fats or with vitamins. A few drops in water before a meal works.

Gamma E Tocopherol/Tocotrienols from Life Extension Foundation

800-544-4440 • *www.lef.org*

Contains all the different fractions of vitamin E for antioxidant effects up to sixty times greater than regular vitamin E.

Moducare Plant Sterolins by New Balance

Plant sterolins have been shown to have a stress hormone and immune response–balance effect.

Silibinin from Life Extension Foundation

800-544-4440 • *www.lef.org*

This potent form of silymarin, the liver-protective and antioxidant component of milk thistle, is the proven liver detoxifier and regenerator I used along with other supportive supplements to reverse my liver illness. Consult a doctor when treating illness.

Venastat by Pharmaton

800-451-6688 • *www.venastat.com*

The key ingredient, an extract from horse-chestnut seed, has been proven to reduce varicose veins and ankle circumference in those with chronic venous insufficiency (varicose veins). Supplements with horse-chestnut-seed extract are available at all vitamin stores.

Probiotics

Acidophilus Pearls™ by Enzymatic Therapy

800-783-2286 • *www.enzy.com*

Advanced "pearl" capsule technology delivers up to 900 percent more live probiotics to the intestine than the leading competitors by protecting the probiotics from stomach acid while in transit.

Natren Healthy Trinity®

www.natren.com

Natren's probiotics have guaranteed potency through a date of expiration. Most other producers guarantee potency at time of manufacture or shipment only. Healthy Trinity contains all three of the most potent super strains of beneficial bacteria. You can find good science-backed information, including probiotic benefits to the skin, on their Web site.

Primal Defense Homeostatic Soil Organisms (HSOs) by Garden of Life

800-622-8986 • *www.gardenoflifeusa.com*

A new generation of probiotics that is thought by some scientists to be more effective in part because they survive heat and do not die off in storage or before they reach the digestive tract.

Skin, Hair, and Nails, Targeted Supplements

Every health supplement affects the skin, but the following supplements offer unique support that can address specific beauty issues more aggressively.

BioSil by Jarrow Formulas

www.jarrow.com

Also available through Life Extension Foundation • 800-544-4440 • *www.lef.org*

This is the most bioavailable form of silicon, which increases collagen content in the dermis.

Diamond Herpanicine

This supplement addresses the viral and immune function that affects outbreaks of cold sores and other skin problems. Contains Lysine and immune-strengthening Astragalus and Echinacea, among other effective herbs.

Enzymatic Therapy

800-783-2286 • *www.enzy.com*

These are high-quality, science-backed supplements like Derma-Klear, Cold Sore Relief, and Hair and Skin Nutrition. Their varicose vein (Varicare) and weight- and hormone-balancing products are powerful.

Injuv®

The first oral hyalouronic acid (HA) supplement may actually build up the skin's inner "moisture sponge"—and do the same for joints. HA is a natural substance that is largely responsible for our ability to hold moisture in the skin and tissues. Available through most vitamin retailers.

Skin, Nails, and Hair DailyFoods by Megafood

800-848-2542 • *www.megafood.com*

This is the only beauty supplement that provides the Foodstate™ , superior form of key supportive nutrients such as silica, sulfur, licorice, and GLA that have been used historically and has been shown in studies to support the skin, nails, and hair. It is far better absorbed than other similar supplements.

Toki by Lane Labs

800-510-2010 • *www.compassionet.com*

Clinical research shows that this lemon-flavored drink increases collagen levels in the blood, and anecdotal evidence is compelling for its effects in plumping up the skin. Takes approximately forty-five days to show effects.

Vivinal two-part nutritional complex for nails

800-318-3934 • *www.viviforyou.com*

This natural marine-protein supplement, in combination with the topically applied myrrh derivative, supports nail strength and may accelerate nail growth.

Viviscal hair and scalp treatments

800-318-3934 • *www.viviforyou.com*

Viviscal showed effectiveness against alopecia areata as well as androgenic hair loss in several published studies. The supplements combined with the topical lotion is most effective. Both contain a marine concentrate, which changes the tissues surrounding the hair follicle, re-establishing the passage of key nutrients required for hair growth.

You're My Everything from Vision, Inc.

888-800-7070 (East Coast) or 888-233-1441 (West Coast) • *www.e3live.com*

Combines the superior form of skin, hair, nail-loving sulfur, MSM, with high-grade powdered blue-green algae and electrolyte sea minerals.

skin care

My criteria for skin products is tough. For maximum results, I've chosen to highlight only products that feature liposome technology, phospholipids, advanced phytonutrients, and marine extracts. Most of the products listed below are made without mineral oil, perfumes, skin-stripping solvents, synthetic colors, and synthetic preservatives. Many of the companies listed below are what I call "microbrews." They are actually microchemists which produce products in small batches that are not warehoused by third parties and that can therefore be delivered fresh and biologically active with the use of little or no preservatives.

A few product categories include synthetics, such as vitamin C serums under "Wrinkles," but my personal feeling is that the benefits of those products outweigh the risks. (Your ultimate criteria should be personal.) That said, I'm always looking for the most natural, pure, or bio-identical formulations and will post them at *www.informedbeauty.com* as they become available. If there's no contact information listed with the product, it is widely available at natural-product and vitamin stores.

Acne and Oily-Skin Products
Acne Soothing Lotion, Neem Oil, and Kapha Essential Oil
by Pratima Skincare
www.pratimaskincare.com
Dr. Pratima Raichur's Ayurvedic Acne Soothing Lotion contains essential oils to heal infections and skin irritations. Neem oil has unique antimicrobial properties, and Kapha Essential Oil blend is designed to balance the Kapha skin type, which is often oily and blemish-prone. (Learn more at her Web site or from her book listed in Suggested Reading.)

Aloe Cleansing Gel by Naturopathica
800-669-7618 • *www.naturopathica.com*
Purifies oily skin without stripping its lipid barrier. Contains no synthetic solvents, petrochemical-derived ingredients, or perfumes.

Balancing Elixir by Zia Natural Cosmetics

800-334-7546 • *www.zianatural.com*

Tea tree, lavender, and clary sage essential oils in a rosemary hydrosol help balance and treat excess oil production. MSM speeds the skin's natural detoxification.

Clearing (Lotion) and Powder Wash by Jules and Jane

www.julesandjane.com

Clearing is a powerful compound including aloe, gotu kola, lavender, willowbark, and zinc that helps heal acne infections and irritations. The Powder Wash is perfect for oily, blemished skin, with Ayurvedic herbs and flower extracts that decongest pores and balance and remineralize the skin. The pure powder form preserves the full potency of the herbs without additives and gently exfoliates with lemon peel, papaya, coriander, sandalwood, and nutmeg.

Grapefruit Complexion Mist by Burt's Bees

www.burtsbees.com

Essential oils of lemon, lime, and grapefruit help balance overactive oil glands, while rosemary helps clear troubled spots. Contains only lime oil, lemon oil, rosemary oil, and grapefruit oil.

Happy Skin Light Box by Verilux

800-786-6850 • *www.verilux.net*

Recent studies in the United Kingdom suggest that isolated red- and blue-light wavelengths help mild to moderate acne by killing bacteria and reducing inflammation. Verilux guarantees results in twelve weeks.

Lotion for Problem Skin with Tea Tree Oil by Arboretum

877-767-9367 • *www.arboretum-skincare.com*

This lotion contains conifer-needle extract, tea tree oil, and Sea Buckthorn oil, and has been shown to have anti-inflammatory and antimicrobial effect and reduce pore size and regulate sebum, while improving the acid-mantle supportive barrier function of the skin with phospholipids

Moss Mask Blemish Remover by Naturopathica

800-669-7618 • *www.naturopathica.com*

Purify blemishes and eliminate redness without destroying the beauty of the skin with potent antibacterial extracts of comfrey, sage, rosemary, chamomile, and moss.

Neroli Toning Serum for Normal and Overactive Skin by Naturopathica

This serum has a base of light apricot-kernel and hazelnut oils. Essential oils of neroli, juniper, and petitgrain keep the skin balanced and help eliminate blackheads and pustules.

Neem Products by Neem Aura Naturals

877-633-6287 • *www.neemaura.com*

Neem's historical use as an antimicrobial, anti-inflammatory, and antifungal is validated in scientific studies. The pure oil and the internal tincture are available through this premiere organic source.

Normalizing Day Oil by Dr. Hauschka

800-247-9907 • *www.drhauschka.com*

Oil can inhibit oil production. This blend contains extracts universally recommended for acne, including St. John's wort and neem, to calm irritation, slow oil production, and refine pores.

Osea Essential Corrective Complex, Acne Spot Treatment

www.oseaskin.com

This super-potent 30 percent essential-oil blend of tea tree, rosemary, grapefruit, lavender, white thyme, and juniper is 100 percent natural and creates a calming, antibacterial, non-drying acne treatment. Cypress may help heal broken capillaries. Vitamin E promotes healing of scarred and damaged skin. Also relieves cold sores and insect bites.

Skin Healing Gel by Youthful Essentials

877-916-1212 • *www.youthfulessentials.com*

Combines carnosine, detoxifying MSM, and vitamin D to speed the healing of skin lesions, acne, burns, and cold sores and to reduce large pores.

Tea Tree Blemish Touch Sticks by Desert Essence

800-439-5506 • *www.mothernature.com*

Contains tea tree oil, which has been shown to work similarly to benzoyl peroxide 5 percent ointments, without the peeling. Also contains skin calmers like calendula, lavender, and anti-inflammatory chamomile. Use five to six times daily for best results.

Zinc Cream by Margarite Cosmetics

800-919-9122 • *www.webvitamins.com*

Fights blemishes and inflammatory skin problems with zinc oxide and sulphur in a tinted base.

Bath and Body Products

Ayurvedic Foot Scrub by Better Botanicals

888-BB-HERBS • *www.betterbotanicals.com*

Everything you desire in a foot scrub. The cooling, antimicrobial effects of eucalyptus, rosemary, and peppermint with the softening, hydrating effects of sea salt and sweet almond oil.

Baby Products

Amikole's Baby Butter

877-576-2825 • *www.sheabutter.net*

Amikole's beautifully packaged blend contains blue chamomile, lavender, melissa, and geranium for a barrier protector, a calming skin effect, and scent.

Desert Essence Baby Talc-Free Powder

800-439-5506 • *www.desertessence.com*

Contains blue cypress to calm irritated skin.

Erbaviva Baby, Pregnancy, and Personal-Care Products

877-372-2848 • *www.erbaviva.com*

The most elegant line I have seen for new babies and their mothers. Gift sets for mothers to be and lavender and oatmeal washing sachets for baby are as beautiful as they are healthful.

Seventh Generation Baby Wipes

Cleanse with pure aloe instead of propylene glycol and synthetic fragrance. Great for removing makeup.

Bath Oil and Shower Gel by Naturopathica

Juniper and Cypress Bath Oil are a wake-up blend to enhance circulation, tone the skin and help the body eliminate toxins. Zesty Lime Shower Gel contains sweet almond protein to maintain the skin's lipid barrier. Extracts of nettle, meadowsweet, and milk thistle hydrate the skin while the lime, blood orange, and ginger intoxicate your senses.

Brown Sugar Body Buff by Zia Natural Cosmetics

800-334-7546 • *www.zianatural.com*

Brown sugar and sea salt, organic clover honey, sea kelp, and algae extracts soften and nourish the skin.

Cardamom Body Sugar by Better Botanicals

With almond, milk, honey, coriander, bitter orange, mandarin, and soy protein, this is sensually out of this world, and a treat for depleted skin.

Cool Mint Body Wash by Terressentials

www.terressentials.com

This is the mint body wash your body's been dreaming of, and the most decadent and potent one you will ever experience. Zero synthetics, and more potent peppermint, spearmint, and other purifying treats than you'll get elsewhere. Feels great all over and is powerful enough to rejuvenate tired, burning feet.

Muti Oils

877-688-4645 • *www.mutioils.com*

100 percent natural aromatherapy products for mothers, pregnant women, babies, and the rest of us. The line includes high-end massage oils, sitz-bath preparations, natural moisturizers with no essential oils for the most sensitive skins, and their popular Uh Oh Migraine Stick.

Olive Oil Soap by Kiss My Face

This 150-year-old formula contains 86 percent olive oil. Going from commercial deodorant body soaps to this soap can make a huge difference in skin health and comfort.

Organic Body Polish, Body Oils, and Body Silks from Trillium Herbal Company

800-734-7253 • *www.trilliumherbal.com*

The Body Polish is made with Pacific sea salt and phospholipid liposomes to hydrate and maintain the skin's lipid barrier, and cold-pressed olive and essential oils such as cedarleaf and rosemary give you amazingly soft skin. The Body Oils, Body Silks, and Body Polishes come in calming, clearing, or warming Ayurvedic herbal blends, as well as an essence-free Body Silk formula for sensitive skin.

Color Cosmetics, High-end Mineral-based

The following cosmetics do not contain coal-tar colors, petrochemicals, or perfumes in their products. All powder mineral makeups have SPF of 18 to 20 and are anti-inflammatory and won't clog the pores. I've highlighted the products that meet the aesthetic demands of the high-end beauty consumer. Every color can be worn anywhere on the face.

Annemarie Borlind

800-447-7024 • *www.borlind.com*

Better foundations, mascaras in beautiful colors like Laguna (a gorgeous turquoise), and gold-tinged, creamy concealers that I use on photo shoots.

Aubrey Organics Natural Lips

1-800-AubreyH • *www.aubrey-organics.com*

Gorgeous colors, colored with beet root and other natural pigments, that I use on photo shoots. I like to mix Natural Red with Mocha for the most rich and complex raisin shade.

Bare Escentuals

800-227-3990 • *www.bareescentuals.com*

This is the widest selection of loose mineral eye shadows, both matte and shimmery. Any color you could want.

Burt's Bees

800-849-7112 • *www.burtsbees.com*

Nice lipsticks, blush creams, and concealers.

Dr. Hauschka

800-247-9907 • *www.drhauschka.com*

These cosmetics are biodynamically produced (the highest form of sustainable agriculture) and elegantly packaged. They offer some great colors and skin formulas. I particularly like the golden peachy blush. Julia Roberts is a Hauschka fan.

Ecco Bella

www.eccobella.com

Beautiful shadow and blush colors. All lipsticks contain organic chamomile, calendula, and jojoba. Flower wax is what makes these products luxurious.

Gabriel Cosmetics

800-439-5506 • *www.mothernature.com*

The glosses, such as Diva, are the perfect nude colors that don't leave you looking washed out. And the gloss really lasts—an impressive feat, especially with no synthetics.

Hemp Organics

877-524-4367 • *www.colorganics.com*

Hemp and castor oil–based lipsticks and lip pencils in great, wearable colors. Vintage Merlot is an amazing blackberry-tinged, juicy burgundy lipstick that has made an impression with models.

Jane Iredale Natural Mineral Cosmetics

800-817-5665 • *www.janeiredale.com*

Recommended by plastic surgeons and makeup artists alike. Powder foundations come in the global, golden tones that truly flatter the skin. The taupe eye pencil and terracotta lip pencils are must-haves. The lip gloss in Melon is a major face brightener I've used for the runway and on photo shoots. Great concealers.

Lavera Natural Cosmetics

877-528-3727 • *www.lavera-usa.com*

This is an elegant line with sophisticated colors, textures, and packaging. Check out the award-winning organic lip glosses that contain berry extracts. Beautiful blue-toned pencils look great on blue eyes.

Youngblood Mineral Cosmetics

www.makeupartistschoice.com

Loose powder pigments and blushes can be mixed into gloss and lip balm for really vibrant color. Brown Sugar and Honey Nut lipsticks and Malt and Mocha lip pencils are staple shades. The foundation-containing pump brush is convenient and portable.

Zia Natural Cosmetics foundation and powders

800-334-7546 • *www.zianatural.com*

Nice gold-tone bronzers and powders.

Zuzu Luxe

If you want a vibrant gloss for spring or even the holiday, try Luscious, a violet-tinged magenta that looks exuberant. It will erase your impression of "dowdy" natural makeup.

Dark Spots and Patches

CamoCare C-Spot Age/Sun Spot Fader

800-CAMOCARE • *www.camocare.com*

Licorice, mulberry root, and Ester-C help fade flat skin spots, discoloration, and freckles.

Skin Answer by Lane Labs

Available from CompassioNet • 800-510-2010

Skin Answer is the only product I know that can eliminate raised, rough sun-damaged spots while leaving healthy skin alone. Requires four to six weeks' daily compliance, and skin will feel irritated—but only the unhealthy tissue—before it is sloughed off. Always have spots checked and supervised by your dermatologist.

Dry-Skin Products

Bio-Hydria Naturesomes by Arbonne International

A phospholipid serum that is applied under moisturizer.

Ceramide Vital Fluid by Annemarie Borlind of Germany

www.borlind.com

This product strengthens the barrier function of the skin. Independent studies showed a significant increase in antioxidant protection and firmness, as well as moisture content and cell generation, without petrochemicals. The fragrance listed is via essential oils, not chemicals.

Evening Primrose Replenishing Eye Cream by Naturopathica

This eye cream contains no waxes—which actually increase puffiness around the eyes. The evening-primrose and borage-seed oils, both high in GLA and anti-oxidants, help rebuild and smooth the driest skin.

Grow Younger Skin Cream by Terra Soleil
A very advanced phospholipid-containing, microbrewed concoction made fresh and delivered directly to you, that carries the purest botanicals, as well as hydrolipid barrier rebuilders, deep into the skin.

Orange Essence Facial Cleanser by Burt's Bees
800-849-7112 • *www.burtsbees.com*
This heavenly smelling, olive oil–based cleanser won an award for its purity and effectiveness. Good for the driest of skins.

Rose and Linden Blossom Face Crème Cleanser by John Masters
Sea-algae extract and plant phospholipids, as well as aloe, sweet-almond protein, ginseng, and vitamins makes this a superior, ultra-gentle cleanser for dry or sensitive skin.

Replinishing Elixir by Zia Natural Cosmetics
800-334-7546 • *www.zianatural.com*
Phospholipids rebuild, MSM aids repair of damaged skin, and neroli hydrosol hydrates.

Skin Food by Weleda
800-241-1030 • *usa.weleda.com*
A pure and live, biodynamically produced cream for super-dry areas that can be applied to body, face, or lips. Contains pansy extract, chamomile, and calendula as well as the finest oils.

See Jing-Jang Crème under "Universal Skin Products."

Inflammatory Skin Problems
Aloe vera gel by Aubrey Organics
800-282-7394 • *www.aubrey-organics.com*
This is the 100 percent pure, real thing. Keep it in the fridge to make it last longer. Great on sunburns.

CamoCare Soothing Cream
800-226-6227 • *www.camocare.com*
Consistent use of this cream may result in the clearing of your rash. The German camillosan chamomile featured in CamoCare products has been shown to be particularly powerful.

Climatotherapy for Psoriasis

To learn more about the proven Dead Sea psoriasis-treatment programs, contact the Dead Sea Research Center (*www.deadsea-health.org*) and the Dead Sea Psoriasis and Arthritis Treatment Foundation (*www.psoriasis-dead-sea.org*).

Earth's Essential Cream by Vision, Inc.

888-800-7070 • *www.e3live.com*

The only truly pure skin cream I have found with healing MSM. This super-rich cream that won't clog pores should replace any petroleum-based heavy or protective creams. Also includes evening-primrose oil (good source of GLA to rebuild lipid barrier and inhibit inflammation), CoQ10, aloe, chamomile, and grapefruit-seed extract, among other antibacterial, antifungal, anti-inflammatory, and cell-regenerative ingredients.

Ecz-cream Oregon Grape Root (Mahonia aquifolium) Cream by Vital Botanicals

800-609-4326 • *www.vitalbotanicals.com*

Helps eczema and other inflammatory skin problems. For even better results, take their Oregon grape root tincture simultaneously, as directed.

Herbacort

800-209-1723 • *www.herbalab.com*

This cream has been formulated to achieve powerful anti-inflammatory effects without steroids.

Licorice Tincture by Herb Pharm

800-223-1216 • *www.vitaminshoppe.com*

To use anti-inflammatory licorice topically, the tincture can be mixed with glycerin or your regular moisturizer applied on its own with a cotton ball to inflamed skin lesions.

Neem Aura Naturals Neem Cream

877-633-6287 • *www.neemaura.com*

Formulated at the highest neem concentration (4 percent) to relieve uncomfortable dry, flaky, chapped, and itchy symptoms of seriously damaged skin.

Penny Island Healing Enzyme-Activated Oat Bath

800-856-1196 • *www.pennyisland.com*

Certified organic colloidal oat bath with proteins and a blend of oat beta glucan forms a moisture barrier and reduces chemically induced irritation.

ThioSkin Zinc Pyrithione Products from ThiOne International, Inc.

www.thione.com

Zinc pyrithione has long been used and recognized for its antifungal and anti-seborrheic effects. More recent studies reconfirmed its power against dandruff. Available in sprays, lotions, and shampoos.

Lip Balms

Green Tea and Mint Lip Balm by Nature's Gate Organics

Contains green tea powder, a potent antioxidant, in a base of nourishing jojoba oil and jojoba wax. Castor-seed oil provides a protective barrier.

Jing Jang Lip Balm

www.jing-jang.com

A cult favorite, this extra-special, comprehensive blend of the best oils, flower extracts, and vitamins makes a truly hydrating, healing, and sealing balm.

Lip Armor by All Terrain

www.allterrainco.com

With unrivaled Z-cote sun protection, shea butter, and high-EFA hemp oil for moisturizing.

Lip Care Balm by Jurlique

800-854-1110 • *www.jurlique.com*

Completely pure, and really fixes dryness. Good to use anywhere on the face to calm and protect dry or peeling patches, such as near the eyebrows or under the nose when you have a cold. A great protective balm for winter.

White Chocolate lip balms by Terressentials

www.terressentials.com

These balms smell and taste unbelievably good, and it's all real. They come in cocoa butter–based White Chocolate Mint (which evokes the Girl Scout cookie favorite) and Orange White Chocolate formulas with vanilla bean. You'll be tempted to lick them off your lips.

Natural Essences and Perfumes

Each of these precious blends and essences will spare you the forty to two hundred or more petrochemical pollutants and aromatic impostors commonly found in synthetic perfumes. Averaging around $20, they also spare your pocketbook.

Aftelier natural perfumes

www.aftelier.com

Elegantly formulated custom solid and liquid natural perfume-essence blends. Celebrated master perfumer Mandy Aftel and her alchemists will create a fragrance personalized for you.

Eau by Jules and Jane

www.julesandjane.com

An androgynously clean, Ayurvedic elixir of prized holy basil, peel of lime, and East Indian sandalwood. No petrochemicals.

Elysian Fields and Angelica Eau de Colognes by Aubrey Organics

800-282-7394 • *www.aubrey-organics.com*

Elysian Fields is a clean, androgynous, woodsy pine-based scent, while Angelica is a mix of wildflower essences.

Essential Oils by Aura Cacia

A few drops of these essential oils can be blended with a teaspoon or more of a carrier oil such as olive, sweet almond, or jojoba for scent, bath, and therapeutic uses.

Florin and Freesia Parfums by Jurlique

800-854-1110 • *www.jurlique.com*

Both of these perfumes are developed from twenty to thirty organic essential oils and resins designed to celebrate purity and beauty.

Perfume With a Purpose by Trillium Herbal Company

www.aromafusion.com

These synergistic roll-on aromatherapy blends feature essences found to have specific effects on mood and mental focus. Love, Work, Play, and Rest blends smell wonderful.

Purifying Purefume Composition by Aveda

800-328-0849 • *www.aveda.com*

This line of Native American spiritual essences features cedar, sage, and sweet grass. Clean and ethereal.

Rosacea and Broken Capillaries

See Happy Skin Light Box under "Acne and Oily-Skin Products."

The blue and red wavelengths address inflammation and bacteria.

Demodicidin Soap and Chang Sheng Soap

800-669-0987 • *www.shoplifestyle.com*

Demodicidin soap may kill the bacteria associated with acne rosacea.

Herbal Celandine Cream by Arboretum Natural Cosmetics

877-767-9367 • *www.arboretum-skincare.com*

An organic, freshly made cream containing celandine and horse-chestnut extracts, potentiated by liposomes to minimize redness and tone and strengthen broken capillaries.

Rosacea Care Serum

www.rosaceacare.com

This is a therapeutic concentration of targeted skin calmers, healers, and rebuilders like phospholipids, willowherb, green tea, vitamin K, glutathione, selenium, and grapeseed.

Rosacea Care Calming Lotion

www.rosaceacare.com

Contains the breakthrough COSMEDERM-7™, a strontium compound proven to block the irritation-producing nerve endings (type C nociceptors) that cause itching, burning, and stinging. The lotion diminishes skin reactivity over time.

Vitamin K Lotion Spray by Orjene Natural Cosmetics

Formulated with vitamin K to help maintain healthy capillaries and pine-needle extract and rice-bran oil to improve the health of skin and underlying tissues.

Scars

Alpha-Lipoic Acid Face Firming Activator with NTP Complex
by N.V. Perricone, M.D., Cosmeceuticals

888-823-7837 • *www.clinicalcreations.com*

Dr. Perricone recommends alpha-lipoic acid for scar-reduction. (See also other products containing alpha-lipoic acid under "Wrinkles.")

Kelocote, Mederma, Laserfade, and other doctor-recommended scar faders

Order from Luminescence • 800-364-6637 • *www.spabeauty.com*

The Skin Store • 888-237-3901 • *www.skinstore.com*

These gels and silicone products sometimes soften scar tissue and flatten raised scars.

Sensitive-Skin Products

Aromessence Rose d'Orient Soothing Concentrate by Decleor

www.sephora.com

A 100 percent pure essential-oil blend specially formulated for sensitive, reactive skin.

Chamomile Cleansing Cream by Naturopathica

800-669-7618 • *www.naturopathica.com*

This therapeutic non-foaming cleanser contains linden flower, ginseng, and German chamomile, known for their soothing properties.

Elemis S.O.S. Emergency Cream

www.elemis.com

This U.K.-based company incorporates precious absolutes, which are the most potent form of essential oils, in their products. This cream calms irritation and sensitivity with lavender, chamomile, eucalyptus, patchouli, myrrh, meadowsweet, willow, and allantoin.

Sun Products

These products feature mineral-based, petrochemical-free sun protection. Micronized zinc oxide is the only substance that offers both UVA and UVB protection, doesn't break down in the sun, and unlike some chemical sunscreens, doesn't accumulate in the body. It is actually anti-inflammatory—which is why it's used in diaper-rash and acne formulas.

All Terrain Performance Sunblocks

www.allterrainco.com

Superior broad-spectrum UVA and UVB protection via Z-Cote in waterproof (AquaSport) and land (TerraSport) formulas. Antioxidants are included for proven added effectiveness. Try the Lip Armor with shea butter and high-EFA hemp-oil moisturizing.

Lavera Family Sun Spray

877-528-3727 • *www.lavera-usa.com*

This innovative product-of-the-year award-winner in 2002 in Europe is a safe, easy-to-apply sunscreen for the whole family.

Sunless Bronze by Annemarie Borlind of Germany

Order from *www.vitaminlife.com*

This sunless tanner imparts a very natural bronze without the petrochemical carriers and perfumes that taint other formulas.

SunSunSun Spray SPF 15 by Annemarie Borlind

www.borlind.com

Advanced skincare and micronized mineral protection against both UVA and UVB rays in a superlight, spray form. Sea buckthorn, rosemary, squalene, vitamin E, and allantoin add additional protection against premature aging and free-radical damage.

Under-Eye Circles

Camocare Gold Under-Eye Therapy

www.abkit.com

With German Camillosan chamomile and alpha lipotene (a form of lipoic acid).

Universal Skin Products

Aromatherapy Eye and Lip Makeup Remover by Reviva Labs

Carrot oil in a base of sweet-almond and wheat-germ oil gives effective and nourishing makeup removal that won't disrupt the lipid barrier of the delicate eye area.

Herbal Extract Recovery Gel by Jurlique

800-854-1110 • *www.jurlique.com*

Deeply hydrates while letting the skin breath. Features powerful antioxidants and anti-inflammatories like chamomile, calendula, echinacea, aloe, green tea, grapeseed, turmeric, and evening-primrose oil. Jurlique's entire line is one of the purest and best. Michelle Pfieffer is an outspoken fan.

Hydrogen Peroxide Instant Oxygen Mask with Green Papaya by Reviva Labs

800-257-7774 • *www.revivalabs.com*

Rather than using alpha-hydroxy acids, use this gentler enzyme-softening mask that doesn't irritate the skin. I use it to prep skin for photo shoots, and the effect is amazing.

Jing-Jang Crème

888-458-3520 • *www.jing-jang.com*

Put this balm anywhere, anytime, to calm, soothe, and protect the skin. Unlike mineral oil or petrolatum, it will not impede skin function. Absolutely the finest calming, hydrating, and healing oils and botanicals go into this deserved cult favorite. No synthetics.

Tea Time Moisturizing Crème by Jason Natural Cosmetics

877-JASON-01 • *www.jason-natural.com*

Every skin type loves this product, which is why it's my official photo-shoot moisturizer. Contains green tea, algae, aloe, squalene, polyphenols, and the super antioxidant S.O.D.

Under Age Ultra Hydrating Moisturizer by Kiss My Face

www.kissmyface.com

A perfect universal moisturizer. Rather than burden the skin with synthetic oils, this fast-penetrating, pre-makeup moisturizer for every skin type contains borage oil, the richest source of GLA, which can rebuild and protect the skin from water loss and inflammation. Organic and free of preservatives, perfumes, and petrochemicals.

Unpetroleum by Avalon Natural Products

www.avalonnaturalproducts.com

The petroleum-jelly alternative with none of the skin function–inhibiting and pore-blocking consequences.

Vitamin K Crème Plus by Jason Natural Cosmetics

877-JASON-01 • *www.jason-natural.com*

Contains the most impressive ingredients I've found in any vitamin K cream, including liposomes, MSM, extracts of horse chestnut and grapeseed, squalane, vitamin C, bioflavanoids, Rosa Mesqueta extract, and bromelain, which has been proven to speed healing. Regular use may improve broken capillaries, redness, under-eye darkness, dry skin, and post-op healing.

The Wonder Cloth

845-342-1009 • *www.wondercloth.com*

This plant fiber and cotton cloth exfoliates gently, removes makeup without remover, and—here's the miracle—rinses stain-free with only water, no matter how much makeup you wipe off with it. I love this cloth and have never found anything else like it.

Varicose Veins

Horse Chestnut Leg Toner by Dr. Hauscka

800-247-9907 • *www.drhauschka.com*

This convenient spray delivers horse-chestnut-bark extract transdermally for better tone.

See Venastat with horse-chestnut seed under "Supplements."

Wrinkles

Bio-Active Marine Complex by Spa Technologies International

800-998-8728 • *www.seaweedproducts..com*

100 percent pure marine algae and protein concentrates transdermally ionize connective tissue to stimulate cell regeneration. More affordable than Crème de La Mer, but with similar ingredients (although La Mer's red algae is said by the company to be specially treated). Demi Moore is a professed fan of this product line, which I find to be outstanding for all skin types.

CoQ10 Facial Cleansing Milk and Perfecting Facial Toner by Avalon Organics

www.avalonnaturalproducts.com

These products contain one of the more comprehensive lineups of antioxidants and skin hydrators, including CoQ10, organic extracts of green tea, ginkgo, echinacea, cucumber, lavender, neroli, aloe, papaya, allantoin, rosemary, sage, and yarrow, as well as panthenol, glycerin, NaPCA, sweet-almond oil, and vitamins E and A. The cleansing milk is a soap-free formula that nourishes rather than depletes. The a lcohol-free toner hydrates and nourishes rather than strips.

Jason Hyper C Serum

800-955-6662 • *www.jason-natural.com*

Although this product doesn't contain the C-Ester form of vitamin C, it is a good high-potency C serum that made a big difference in my skin.

Suis Anti-Aging Serum

888-237-3901 • *www.skinstore.com*

Contains a seaweed polysaccharide complex, which will give you plump, smooth skin without alpha-hydroxy acids. Can be used during the day under moisturizer.

Vitamin C and A Ultra Rich Moisturizer by Kiss My Face

www.kissmyface.com

For the purist, vitamins C-ester (ascorbyl palmitate), E, and A in a GLA-rich, skin-regenerating organic formula with green tea and grapeseed oil and zero synthetics. Rich without being heavy. Absorbs completely, so it's great over serums. No preservatives, oils, or perfumes. Real rose and honeysuckle smell heavenly.

Vitamin C-Ester/DMAE/Alpha Lipoic Acid Products

These products are based on Dr. Perricone's research on C-Ester, the more stable, less irritating form of fat-soluble vitamin C. Used daily, these products will reduce wrinkles and make the skin more radiant. Few of the vitamin C serums are completely natural, but the benefits may outweigh the negatives here. Those who are extremely sensitive may want to check the ingredients and decide accordingly. Use these products at night, with or without moisturizer.

Alpha Lipoic Acid, Vitamin C Ester, and DMAE cream by Reviva Labs

www.revivalabs.com

Contains the above key ingredients, plus soy phospholipid liposome delivery, in one of the more natural formulations.

Age Eraser with Kinetin by Age Advantage Laboratories

888-833-3511 • *www.ageadvantagelabs.com*

Kinetin works comparably to Retin A, Renova, and alpha-hydroxy acids without the peeling and sun-vulnerability side effects. This is one of the most impressive Kinetin products I've found.

High Potency Vitamin C-Ester Serum by Age Advantage Laboratories
888-833-3511 • *www.ageadvantagelabs.com*
The C-Ester Serum offers high-potency effects and deep transdermal delivery with the aid of emu oil. This serum can be used with the Age Eraser with Kinetin.

C-Ester, DMAE and Alpha Lipoic Acid products by Dr. Nicholas Perricone
888-823-7837 • *www.clinicalcreations.com*
Use with the corresponding supplements for augmented benefits.

Skin Eternal Serum by Source Naturals
www.sourcenaturals.com
These serums contain CoQ10, MSM, and vitamins A, D3, and E. Take their Skin Eternal Tablets for greater effect.

Youthful Essentials Wrinkle Serum
877-916-1212 • *www.youthfulessentials.com*
The only 100 percent natural C-Ester serum I've found, and the only one containing a high potency of carnosine, the remarkable anti-aging substance, along with the other skin stars, alpha-lipoic acid, DMAE, vitamins A and E, MSM, and green tea extracts.

See Injuv and Toki under "Supplements."

hair products

Cleansers and Conditioners, Non-stripping
These shampoos contain no sulfates and are packed with the world's most amazing substances.

Extra Light and Deep Conditioning Hair Oils by Urban Botanica
www.urbanbotanica.com
Extra Light Hair Oil contains virgin grapeseed, sweet almond, jojoba, geranium, and citrus oil for ultra-light gloss and control. The Deep Conditioning Hair Oil contains virgin coconut oil and vanilla essential oil blended with avocado butter and herbs.

Herbal Hair and Scalp Conditioner (Pomade) by Urban Botanica
www.urbanbotanica.com
A scalp and hair treatment and styling pomade in one. Free of petrochemicals and beeswax, which can build up. Feeds your head with nothing but mango and shea butters and avocado and coconut oils.

Lemon Verbena Clarifying Shampoo by Avalon Organic Botanicals
Use every other week to remove product residue. It's also great for detoxing your hair before starting to use non-foaming cleansers, and periodically thereafter.

Pure Earth Hair Wash by Terressentials
This non-foaming aromatic wash containing organic shavegrass, natural clay minerals, nettle, rose geranium, and other scalp-clarifying and -stimulating extracts absorbs a bit more oil than the Wen Cleanser and may be better for oilier hair. As your hair detoxes its synthetic buildup, your mane will feel much softer.

Shampoos, Rinses, and Detanglers by John Masters Organics
www.johnmasters.com
Masters's products are among the highest-end organic hair products available. With regular clients like Sarah Jessica Parker and Winona Ryder, they have to be. Evening Primrose Shampoo is one of the only shampoos for dry hair that actually moisturizes the hair. Citrus and Neroli Detangler conditions weightlessly. Herbal Cider Hair Rinse and Clarifier removes buildup and restores proper pH to hair and scalp. Lavender and Avocado Intensive Conditioner quenches the driest hair.

Wen Conditioning Cleansers
www.chazdeanstudio.com
This formula, created by celebrated hair stylist Chaz Dean, doesn't lather up, softens the hair on contact, and rinses out completely. People with dry, coarse hair that gets big after washing will love this product.

Dandruff
Zinc and Sage Shampoo with Conditioner by John Masters Organics
www.johnmasters.com
A great alternative to synthetic dandruff shampoos, this will help diminish itching and flaking.

ThioSkin Shampoo

www.thione.com

A shampoo containing zinc pyrithione that offers proven benefits with a less synthetic, more therapeutic formula than standard dandruff shampoos.

Hair Color

The pickings for nontoxic hair color are slim. The ones available at the health-food stores still contain phenylenediamine-related chemicals, even if in lower concentrations. Doing a foil-weave instead of an overall color or going lighter instead of darker are two ways to ease the toxic burden.

Logona Herbal Hair Colors

800-648-6654 • *www.logona.co.uk*

Unlike other so-called natural hair colors, this one really contains none of the cancer-linked phenylenediamine or its sister chemicals.

Hair-Loss Formulas

Hair regrowth without drugs is a joyful reality, but the process takes at least three months to merely stop hair loss, another few months to show regrowth, and up to nine months to fully restore the hair. Be patient and consistent.

Hair Genesis

800-736-0729 • *www.hairgenesis.com*

Hair Genesis, a DHT-inhibiting formula, works as well as prescription hair-loss drugs without the side effects.

Hair Regrowth Formula by Dr. Peter Proctor

Order from 800-544-4440 • *www.lef.org*

Dr. Proctor, a noted hair-loss researcher, developed Hair Regrowth Shampoo and other formulas based on a compound called NANO (3-carboxylic acid pyridine-N-oxide), which he refers to as "natural" minoxidil. It works.

Nu Hair with Shen Min and Saw Palmetto

www.nuhair-hair-loss-balding-treatment.com

In addition to proven DHT-inhibiting saw palmetto, Nu Hair contains fo-ti, also known as he shou wu, which is prescribed widely in Chinese traditional medicine to combat premature aging and graying hair.

Revivogen

888-616-HAIR • *www.revivogen.com*

Revivogen contains other promising DHT-inhibiting substances such as zinc and azelaic acid.

Viviscal

800-318-3934 • *www.viviforyou.com*

Viviscal shows effectiveness against alopecia areata as well as androgenic hair loss.

Styling and Texturizing

Chi Air Ceramic, Ionic, Infrared Professional Hair Dryer

877-923-3400 • *www.webbeautystore.com*

Ionic and infrared blow-dryers dry hair in half the time without damage, because they use a different kind of heat that evenly penetrates and does not scorch the hair. This is the handsomest, high-end professional dryer to combine ionic and infrared technology. A wise—though expensive—investment in healthier hair, especially if you blow-dry often.

Ion Shine Hair Dryer by Conair

Order from Lifestyle Fascination • 800-669-0987

Less expensive than the Chi Air dryer.

Jason Fresh Botanicals Hairspray

Contains no PVP (a common ingredient in hairsprays that causes buildup, drying out the hair as well as flaking). Amino acids, soy and wheat proteins give body as glycerin, yarrow, cherry bark, and natural gums give a hydrated, flexible hold. I like to spray it on my fingers and rake them through the hair for texture that looks wild but stays.

Maniatis Quick-dry Hair Towel through CCB-Paris

800-758-1337

This hair chamois minimizes blow-drying time.

MOP Pomade

866-699-4667 • *www.mopproducts.com*

Although I use this product on photo shoots all the time to control and defrizz coarse, wavy hair, it is intended to maintain straight hair by blocking humidity. It's a great waxy, shine-enhancing product that utilizes castor oil and beeswax, organic hops, nettle, and lemongrass instead of sebum-blocking mineral oil or petrolatum-based pomades.

Primrose Tangle-Go Conditioner, Lusterizer, and Styling Spray by Aubrey Organics

800-AubreyH • *www.aubrey-organics.com*

A really great lusterizer for styling or moisturizing the hair at the beach.

Texturizer, Defrizzer Serum, and Pomade by John Masters Organics

www.johnmasters.com

The blood-orange and bourbon-vanilla Texturizer is a versatile styling delicacy for the hair and the senses. The Defrizzer offers light control, without impeding the therapeutic action of sebum as silicone serums can. The Hair Pomade with organic mango butter and babassu oil controls and shapes short styles and frizzy hair and makes a great elbow, heel, and cuticle balm.

Weleda Rosemary Hair Oil

800-241-1030 • *usa.weleda.com*

A delicacy for dry hair. Rub a few drops into the palms and then into damp or dry hair for sheen and an incredible scent.

Wild Lime Hair Polish by Aesop

Order from CosmetiqueBeauty • 800-892-5320

Scented with West Indian wild limes, this product adds body to and protects fine, flat, or limp hair. A dab can be used on wet or dry hair, with or without styling tools.

nail products

Firoze Professional Nail Polish

866-866-1316 • *www.firoze.com*

The only professional-quality nail polish free of the top three dangerous nail-polish chemicals: formaldehyde, toluene, and dibutyl phthalate.

Non-Toxic Nail Polishes and Polish Remover by Earthly Delights

800-643-4221 • *www.internatural-alternative-health.com*

These water-based nail polishes—any color, including foil metallics—look good but don't last as long as the Firoze. The acetone-free, non-toxic Naked Nails nail-polish remover has zero chemical smell, moisturizes the nail, and removes the toughest polish, including glitter polish.

NonyX Nail Gel

Order from Swanson Health Products • *www.swansonvitamins.com*

This nontoxic gel containing naturally derived ethanoic acid can clear nail fungus and restore normal nail growth in about twelve months, even if you've had fungus all your life.

Vivinal Nail Growth Accelerator and Strengthener

800-318-3934 • *www.viviforyou.com*

This product contains nothing but 100 percent pure myrrh derivative, which has been shown to dramatically thicken nails and support nail growth, particularly when taken with the supporting Vivinal Marine Protein Complex supplements.

bathroom-cabinet products

Cold Sores

ViraMedx Cold Sore Medication

800-224-4024 • *www.viramedx.com*

The only cold-sore medication—natural or otherwise—shown in published studies to give substantial and consistent healing in twenty-four hours, even against drug-resistant outbreaks.

See Diamand Herpanicine under "Skin, Hair, and Nails, Targeted Supplements."

Deodorants

Natural deodorants are about finding what works with your chemistry.

Dr. Hauschka Deodorants

800-247-9907 • *www.drhauschka.com*

Containing zinc ricinoleate, these deodorants inhibit bacteria that cause odor without interfering with the important function of perspiration.

Lavilin

This is one of the strongest natural deodorants, but it's very expensive.

Herbal Clear and Nature's Gate Organics Deodorants

Unlike other stick deodorants, these are propylene-glycol (PG)free. Also free of aluminum, the Herbal Clear with Hidrox® uses powerful antimicrobials from olive and lichen. Nature's Gare uses essential oils.

Weleda Sage

This one worked far better for me than most natural deodorants, and it smells incredible. It doubles as an androgynous, long-lasting scent.

Insect Repellent

Herbal Armor Outdoor Protection by All Terrain Company, Inc.

www.allterrainco.com

This is the only high-tech natural insect repellent that is sub-micron-encapsulated for time-released delivery of proven insect-repelling essential oils. Carries none of the risks of DEET. Also available with SPF 15 from Z-cote.

Mouth-care Products

Kiss My Face AloeDyne Fresh Breath Mouthwash

www.kissmyface.com

With organic aloe, vitamin K, tea tree oil, grapefruit seed extract, and horse chestnut—a stellar list.

Zap Breath Strips by Nature's Gate

Order from Levlad, Inc. • 800-327-2012 • *www.levlad.com*

Made with green tea, these strips are the truly fresh alternative to synthetically flavored, colored, and produced breath strips.

Calendula and Plant Gel Toothpaste by Weleda

800-241-1030 • *www.weleda.com*

Myrrh, licorice root, and clove oil offer proven gum health and anti-inflammatory benefits.

XyliChew by Tundre Trading Inc.

800-439-5506 • *www.mothernature.com*

Xylitol-sweetened gum prevents tooth decay and inhibits mouth bacteria.

Oral Comfort Toothpaste and Mouthwash Spray
by Jason Natural Cosmetics
www.jason-natural.com

Powerful antimicrobial grapefruit-seed extract, aloe, proven decay-inhibitor xylitol, tissue-healer MSM, parsley extract, and gum-healer CoQ10 make a stellar toothpaste. The mouthwash spray contains the above ingredients, along with powerful anti-bacterial oregano oil, zinc, green tea, and cranberry. I have not found better mouthcare products in my search.

Gary Null's Clean Teeth

Top gum healers like myrrh extract, eucalyptus oil, clove oil, and proven decay-inhibiting xylitol, as well as infection-fighting echinacea, organic tea tree oil, aloe, healing calendula, and bloodroot make an amazing toothpaste.

Tongue Brush by Enfresh
www.enfresh.com

A gentle, short-bristled brush that easily gives you a new way to reach the back of the tongue, where much of the odor-causing bacteria dwell. More pleasant to use than tongue scrapers. I use it with the Jason Oral Comfort Mouthwash Spray.

Nasal and Sinus Products
NasalCrom Allergy Prevention

877-925-5374 • *www.nasalcrom.com*

These products have been proven to prevent and relieve nasal allergic symptoms without side effects. Available at most drug stores.

Xlear Nasal Wash

877-599-5327 • *www.xlear.com*

Shown to inhibit bacteria adherence and reduce or halt sinus infections.

Zicam Nasal Gel

877-942-2626 • *www.zicam.com*

Proven to stop sinus infections in their tracks and to reduce the duration of the common cold without side effects. Available at drug stores and health-food stores.

Sleep Products

Anti-allergy dust-mite-barrier bedding

Order from Gaiam • 877-989-6321 • *www.gaiam.com*

Can help you wake up without the puffy under-eye circles and other allergy symptoms.

Silent Snore

www.silentsnore.com

Sprayed to the back of the throat and then swallowed, this product stopped or reduced snoring in 90 percent of people tested in a clinical trial. Similar products work by reducing swelling and blockage in the back of the throat.

Sleep Bedtime Balm by Essence of Vali

www.essenceofvali.com

Essential oils such as lavender have demonstrated sedative effects in several studies. Balms are applied directly to the upper lip. This award-winning balm is formulated to reduce anxiety and can be used conveniently and portably at any time, unlike diffusers.

The Big Guns

Each of these valuable products, except Xlear, is available at health-food stores.

Cranactin Cranberry Capsules by Solaray

Great for preventing bladder infections.

Nutribiotic GSE products

Available in liquid, capsules, ear drops, foot sprays, deodorants, and dental products, these products feature GSE's powerful antimicrobial action.

Oregano Oil by North American Herb and Spice

800-243-5242

This powerful antimicrobial killed strep and Candida albicans in test-tube studies. You can get it in tincture and capsule form. It's really strong, so be sure to dilute it. Always work with your doctor if you're fighting an illness.

Sambucol Elderberry Syrup

Elderberry has been proven to fight flu symptoms.

Tea tree oil products by Desert Essence and Thursday Plantation

Oral care, foot products, and deodorants, as well as dental, hair, skin, and blemish treatments are available.

Xlear Nasal Wash

www.xlear.com

Not widely available, this nasal wash, as well as other products containing xylitol, which has been shown to inhibit oral, nasal, and middle-ear infections, is a valuable staple.

Zand Formula Echinacea and Goldenseal Tincture

www.zand.com

These ingredients are proven to boost immunity and fight infection.

home appliances

Aquaspace Water Filtering Carafe

800-705-5559

Unlike other pitcher-type filters that affect taste and sediment, this pitcher removes more than forty-five volatile organic chemicals, including cryptosporidium, and the filter lasts more than ten times as long.

Miracle Juicer from Phillips Products and Services

800-705-5559

Deemed one of the most efficient and durable juicers for the money by many top practitioners.

Multi-Pure Water Filters

800-622-9206

One of the best water purifiers out there.

Nikken Water Filters

Order from *www.informedbeauty.com* and other distributors. These are magnetized and alkalizing sink, shower, and portable, high-end, water-bottle filters that increase water penetration into the tissues and alkalize the body. More expensive than standard filters.

Shower Filters using zinc-copper technology

A variety of these filters are available through *www.gaiam.com*.

Sonicare Toothbrush

www.sonicare.com

Uses sonic waves, widely recommended by doctors and dentists for its ability to inhibit bacteria below the gumline and discourage canker sores.

Sun Pure Air purifier

800-705-5559

Uses UV against germs and HEPA, carbon, and xeolite, which eliminate particles, chemicals, gases, and odors.

Vita-Mix Super 5000

800-VITAMIX • *www.vitamix.com*

The only machine that not only makes sorbets, hummus, and soups but also grinds flour and seeds. For free shipping through my Web site, *www.informedbeauty.com*, use code ITKJA02.

mail-order and on-line catalogs and services

Gaiam

877-989-6321 • *www.gaiam.com*

A holistic lifestyle source for personal-care products, organic clothing and bedding, unbleached paper and feminine hygiene products, nontoxic household cleaners, yoga and fitness products, mind/body/spirit books, solar-powered products, water and air purifiers, and great gifts.

Cutting Edge Catalog

800-497-9516 • *www.cutcat.com*

Water and air purifiers, full-spectrum lighting, Chromalux lightbulbs, electro-magnetic field (EMF) computer and cell-phone shields, and therapeutic light boxes.

Life Extension Magazine

800-544-4440 • *www.lef.org*

This stellar publication put out by the nonprofit Life Extension Foundation is educational and a mail-order resource for some of the best supplements available—and for learning which studies have been done on them. You can even order personal blood testing.

Swanson Health Products

800-437-4148 • *www.swansonvitamins.com*

This company offers affordable and harder-to-find supplements.

The Vitamin Shoppe

800-223-1216 • *www.vitaminshoppe.com*

Offers an endless array of most of the reputable brand-name supplements, natural personal-care products, specialty teas and foods (such as some of the low-carb brands listed under "Foods and Beverages"). Its Web site offers an easy-to-use *Healthnotes* database to look up specific supplements, health issues, and published research.

Health-Testing Services

ALCAT Delayed Food Allergy Testing

800-881-2685 ext. 107 • *www.alcat.com*

Considered to be the most accurate and sensitive test for food sensitivities.

Blood-Testing Services through Life Extension Foundation

800-544-4440 • *www.lef.org*

State-of-the-art testing is offered directly to consumers from top labs all over the country. Have your DHEA, hormone levels, homocysteine, and other health issues tested.

organizations, educational resources, and services

AlternativeMedicine.com

1650 Tiburon Boulevard, Tiburon, CA 94920

800-515-4325 • *www.alternativemedicine.com*

The Internet's largest database of alternative medical information. Join informative communities for specific health concerns and search the database for alternative practitioners and health-food stores in your neck of the woods.

American Association for Health Freedom

9912 Georgetown Pike, Suite D-2; P.O. Box 458, Great Falls, VA 22066

800-230-2762; fax 703-759-6711

info@healthfreedom.net • www.healthfreedom.net

An organization of healthcare practitioners who use nutritional and other complementary therapies. The AAHF Web site provides a directory of member practitioners to help you find a good doctor near you.

The American Academy of Environmental Medicine

7701 East Kellogg, Suite 625, Wichita, KS 67207

316-684-5500; fax 316-684-5709

administrator@aaem.com • www.aaem.com

A medical society of clinicians who take a proactive and preventive approach to addressing the environmental causes of illnesses. Physicians listed in the directory are certified to have completed training and have passed the board examination for environmental medicine.

American Association of Naturopathic Physicians (AANP)

3201 New Mexico Avenue NW, Suite 350, Washington, DC 20016

866-538-2267; fax 202-274-1992

member.services@naturopathic.org • www.naturopathic.org

An organization of physicians dedicated to promoting the effective use of natural therapies. A directory of member physicians is available on its Web site.

The American Botanical Council (ABC)

6200 Manor Road, Austin, TX 78723

512-926-4900; fax 512-926-2345

abc@herbalgram.org • www.herbalgram.org

The American Botanical Council publishes information on the safe and effective use of medicinal plants and phytomedicines. The ABC Web site provides free information on common herbs, as well as more extensive information to ABC members, including an on-line version of the German Commission E Monographs—Therapeutic Guide to Herbal Medicines.

American College for the Advancement of Medicine (ACAM)

23121 Verdugo Drive, Suite 204, Laguna Hills, CA 92653

800-532-3688; fax 949-455-9679 • *www.acam.org*

ACAM is a nonprofit medical society dedicated to educating physicians and other healthcare professionals on the latest in preventive/nutritional medicine. Access its listing of alternative physicians in the United States on its Web site.

Beyond Pesticides

National Coalition Against the Misuse of Pesticides

701 E Street SE, #200, Washington, DC 20003

202-543-5450; fax 202-543-4791

info@beyondpesticides.org • *www.beyondpesticides.org*

Go here for information on pesticides and alternatives to their use.

Broda O. Barnes, M.D., Research Foundation, Inc.

P.O. Box 110098, Trumbull, CT 06611

203-261-2101; fax 203-261-3017

info@brodabarnes.org • *www.brodabarnes.org*

A key source for thyroid diagnosis and treatment information.

Burzynski Clinic and Burzynski Research Institute

9432 Old Katy Road, Suite 200, Houston, TX 77055

713-335-5697; fax 713-335-5699 • *www.cancermed.com*

Dr. Burzynski's groundbreaking cancer treatment has shown a high success rate with brain tumors.

The Cancer Prevention Coalition, Inc. (CPC)

c/o School of Public Health, University of Illinois at Chicago

2121 West Taylor Street, MC 922, Chicago, IL 60612

312-996-2297 • *www.preventcancer.com*

A unique nationwide coalition of leading independent experts in cancer prevention and public health, together with citizen activists, with a shared mission to reduce escalating cancer rates through public education.

Complementary Alternative Medical Association

cama@camaweb.org • www.camaweb.org

A medical-freedom organization promoting the practice of complementary and alternative medicine and consumer control over healthcare choices.

Citizens for Health

5 Thomas Circle NW, Suite 500, Washington, DC 20009

info@citizens.org • www.citizens.org

A nonprofit, grassroots, consumer-advocacy group that champions public policies empowering individuals to make informed health choices. This group depends on your membership and donations.

Co-op America

1612 K Street NW, Suite 600, Washington, DC 20006

800-58-GREEN; fax 202-331-8166 • *www.coopamerica.org*

Here you'll learn about which corporations are benefiting people and which are harming them and the environment and how to buy and invest in harmony with your values.

The Consumers Union

101 Truman Avenue, Yonkers, NY 10703-1057

914-378-2000; fax 914-378-2928 • *www.consumersunion.org*

This is the publisher of *Consumer Reports* magazine and an independent nonprofit testing, educational, and information organization serving only the consumer.

The Environmental Health Network

P.O. Box 1155, Larkspur, CA 94977

415-541-5075 • *www.ehnca.org*

An organization for people with environmental-chemical concerns and sensitivities.

Fairness and Accuracy in Reporting (FAIR)

112 W. 27th Street, New York, NY 10001

212-633-6700; fax 212-727-7668

fair@fair.org • www.fair.org

A national media-watch group that has been offering well-documented criticism of media bias and censorship since 1986.

Foundation for the Advancement of Innovative Medicine (FAIM)

Two Executive Boulevard, Suite 206, Suffern, NY 10901

877-634-3246 • *faim@healthlobby.com* • *www.faim.org*

FAIM provides "a voice for innovative medicine's professionals, patients, and suppliers" and defines "innovative medicine" as therapy that has been shown to have clinical value yet is outside the mainstream of conventional medicine. The FAIM Web site has a directory of member clinicians. Members receive a health newsletter and receive discounts from selected suppliers.

Glycemic Index Online

www.glycemicindex.com

The University of Sydney's GI Web site provides information on the GI of foods, latest GI data, new research, GI books, GI testing services, and information on the GI symbol program.

HealthWorld Online

4049 Lyceum Avenue, Los Angeles, CA 90066 • *www.healthy.net*

This virtual health village provides a wide range of information, products, and services to help consumers create and manage a wellness-based lifestyle. Click on "Find a Professional" to find a complementary physician near you.

Herb Research Foundation

1007 Pearl Street, Suite 200, Boulder, CO 80302

www.herbs.org

A great resource for information on herbs and their proven effects. The Herb Research Foundation's custom research service provides affordable custom searches for literature on herbs.

The IDentity Project

P.O. Box 5545, Atlanta, GA 31107-0545

P.O. Box 14958, Cincinnati, OH 45250-0958

888-415-5418 • *info@identityproject.org* • *www.identityproject.org*

Produced by "Communicating the Power of One," this organization offers information on eating-disorder awareness and body-image empowerment.

Life Extension Foundation (LEF)

P.O. Box 229120, Hollywood, FL 33022

Orders 800-544-4440; 954-766-8433; fax 954-761-9199

www.lef.org

Arguably the best single professional- and consumer-friendly source for information on combining conventional and proven alternative therapies. This organization has historically broken medical news ten or more years before the mainstream. Call or visit its Web site to find out more about membership, supplements, and its magazine. Sign your doctor up, too.

Local Harvest

www.localharvest.org

Use this site to find an organic farmer near you.

National Center for Complementary and Alternative Medicine (NCCAM) at the National Institutes of Health (NIH)

NCCAM Clearinghouse

P.O. Box 7923, Gaithersburg, MD 20898-7923

888-644-6226; fax 866-464-3616

info@nccam.nih.gov • nccam.nih.gov

NCCAM is the NIH effort to sponsor rigorous research on complementary and alternative medicine and to keep up with domestic studies of alternative therapies.

The National Institutes of Health (NIH)

9000 Rockville Pike, Bethesda, MD 20892

301-496-4000 • *nihinfo@od.nih.gov • www.nih.gov*

NIH provides access to information and help on all kinds of health issues, including addictions. Toll-free information lines are listed at *www.nih.gov/health/infoline.htm*.

The National Nutritional Foods Association

3931 MacArthur Boulevard, Suite 101, Newport Beach, CA 92660-3013

800-966-6632; fax 949-622-6266

nnfa@nnfa.org • www.nnfa.org

An organization that fights for our continued access to supplements and healthy food.

The New Zealand Dermatological Society

www.dermnetnz.org

This award-winning Web site offers graphic pictures and details about any skin disorder to help you identify mysterious skin problems and rashes.

Organic Consumer's Association (OCA)

6101 Cliff Estate Road, Little Marais, MN 55614

218-226-4164; fax 218-353-7652 • *www.organicconsumers.org*

The OCA, a key organization in upholding environmentally crucial agricultural methods, sponsors campaigns to support the use of organic and sustainable agriculture. A great resource for news, it provides directories of natural-food stores, farmers markets, and the like.

Public Interest Research Groups (PIRG)

218 D Street SE, Washington, DC 20003

202-546-9707; fax 202-546-2461 • *www.pirg.org*

The Public Interest Research Groups are an alliance of state-based, citizen funded organizations dedicated to uncovering threats to public health and well-being and fighting to end them. Its mission is to deliver persistent, result-oriented activism that protects the environment, encourages a fair marketplace for consumers, and fosters responsive, democratic government.

PubMed on Medline

www.pubmed.org

This is the database your doctor relies on, though it is unlikely that he or she does much searching on natural therapies. You can access free indexed medical literature from the vast Medline database through the National Institutes of Health (NIH). Just type in your condition or the substance or drug you want information on.

Talk Surgery, Inc.

33 Prince Street, Suite 304, Montreal, Quebec H3C 2M7 Canada

866-875-8255; fax 514-875-1214

www.talksurgery.com/consumer/procedures/skin_treatments.html

This link provides a community where you can read firsthand accounts of individuals' experiences with laser and light skin-treatment information.

Total Transformation Programs

programs@informedbeauty.com • www.informedbeauty.com

Kat James's land- and sea-based experiential programs, where participants experience the dawn-to-dusk principles and results of the process of shedding.

Union of Concerned Scientists

2 Brattle Square, Cambridge, MA 02238-9105

617-547-5552; fax 617-864-9405 • *www.ucsusa.org*

A group of scientists who can't be bought have formed a coalition to inform the public of science so they can be involved in decisions that affect their health and the future of the planet.

USDA's Alternative Farming Systems Information Center

10301 Baltimore Avenue, Room 132, Beltsville, MD 20705-2351

301-504-6559; fax 301-504-6409

afsic@nal.usda.gov • www.nal.usda.gov/afsic

AFSIC specializes in locating and accessing information related to alternative cropping systems, including sustainable, organic, low-input, biodynamic, and regenerative agriculture. Visit *www.nal.usda.gov/afsic/csa/csastate.htm* to find an alternative farm near you.

newsletters and periodicals

These newsletters can help one stay five or more years ahead of the curve without reading medical journals. These are among the best existing resources for staying informed. The information is not based on economic relevance but on what really works.

Alternative Medicine magazine

1650 Tiburon Boulevard, Tiburon, CA 94920

800-515-4325 • *www.alternativemedicine.com*

Offers information on herbs, supplements, and other natural therapies as well as on natural beauty and household products.

Better Nutrition magazine

www.betternutrition.com

Informs readers on the latest breakthroughs in nutritional approaches to optimal health and ongoing research into vitamins, botanicals (herbs), minerals and other supplements. Available at health-food and natural products stores. Find which stores near you carry it by logging on to its Web site.

Dr. Jonathan V. Wright's *Nutrition and Healing*

702 Cathedral Street, Baltimore, MD 21201

800-851-7100 • *www.wrightnewsletter.com*

Dr. Wright is one of the most peer-respected pioneers and authorities on alternatives.

Dr. Stephen Sinatra's *The Sinatra Health Report*

Advanced Bio Solutions

Customer Service Center

P.O. Box 52, Arden, NC 28704

888-887-7498 • *www.drsinatra.com*

A monthly newsletter focused on tips for increased longevity and quality of life.

The Health Sciences Institute Members Alert

Health Sciences Institute

702 Cathedral Street, Baltimore, MD 21201

800-981-7157 • *www.hsibaltimore.com*

A cutting-edge newsletter put out by a stellar editorial board of top medical experts. Here you will learn many facts before you hear them anywhere else.

Dr. Julian Whitaker's *Health and Healing*

7811 Montrose Road, Potomac, MD 20854

800-539-8219 • *www.drwhitaker.com*

Dr. Whitaker is not only a medical pioneer but a freedom of speech hero.

Dr. David Williams's *Alternatives*

7811 Montrose Road, Potomac, MD 20854

800-527-3044 • *www.drdavidwilliams.com*

You'll learn many facts in this newsletter years before they hit mainstream.

Dr. Susan M. Lark's *The Lark Letter: A Woman's Guide to Optimal Health and Balance*

7811 Montrose Road, Potomac, MD 20854-3394

800-829-5876 • *www.drlark.com*

Dr. Lark is a champion for women's health. Get this newsletter for great information on hormone-related weight issues and other health issues.

Healthnotes

1505 SE Gideon Street, Suite 200, Portland, OR 97202

800-659-7630 • *info@healthnotes.com* • *www.healthnotes.com/consumer/*

A leading provider of highly referenced, user-friendly alternative health information that can be accessed through in-store touch-screen kiosks and the Web sites of several major vitamin and natural-product retailers.

HerbalGram

American Botanical Council

6200 Manor Road, Austin, TX 78723

512-926-4900; fax 512-926-2345 • *www.herbalgram.org/herbalgram/*

A top educational resource on herbs published by the American Botanical Council.

Dr. Christiane Northrup's *Health Wisdom for Women*

800-804-0935 • *www.drnorthrup.com*

A must-read if you're facing menopausal issues and want to explore emotional connections with disease.

Life Extension Magazine

Life Extension Foundation

P.O. Box 229120, Hollywood, FL 33022

Orders 800-544-4440; 954-766-8433 • *www.lef.org*

This is perhaps the most cutting-edge, authoritative health resource I've found. Become a member and get the magazine. Log on for medical abstracts and protocols to show your doctor. This organization saves lives and helps to preserve our medical freedom.

Rachel's Environment and Health Weekly
Environmental Research Foundation
P.O. Box 160, New Brunswick, NJ 08903-0160
888-272-2435; fax 732-791-4603
erf@rachel.org • *www.rachel.org*
Named in honor of Rachel Carson, author of *Silent Spring*, this is a free electronic newsletter on toxic substances and other environmental hazards published by the Environmental Research Foundation.

Total Health Magazine
165 North 100 East. Ste. 2, St. George, UT 84770
888-316-6051 • *www.totalhealthmagazine.com*
Always offers the knowledge of a variety of the most informed experts, I highly recommend this magazine.

suggested reading

The most valuable health resources for you and your family are those that will resonate with your doctor via peer-reviewed, published studies but which at the same time are presented in a way that laymen can easily use and understand. The following resources meet this tough criterion and will put you light-years ahead of the general public in terms of usable quality-of-life choices. I highly recommend that you use several of them the next time you or a loved one has a health concern. And you may want to offer a second copy as a gift to the skeptical conventional physician in your life. Most of these books can be ordered from *www.informedbeauty.com*.

Aesoph, Lauri, M.D. *Your Natural Health Makeover*. New York: Prentice Hall, 1998.

Atkins, Robert C., M.D. *Dr. Atkins' New Diet Revolution*. New York: HarperCollins, 1992, 1999, 2002.

Balch, James F., M.D., and Phyllis A. Balch, C.N.C. *Prescription for Nutritional Healing*, 3rd ed. New York: Avery Penguin Putnam, 2000.

Blaylock, Russell L., M.D. *Excitotoxins: The Taste That Kills*. Santa Fe, N.M.: Health Press, 1997.

Blumenthal, Mark, Josef Brinckman, and Alicia Goldberg. *Herbal Medicine: Expanded Commission E Monographs*. Boston: Integrative Medicine Communication, 2000.

Bradshaw, John. *Bradshaw on the Family: A New Way of Creating Self-Esteem*. Deerfield Beach, Fla.: Health Communications, 1996.

Brand-Miller, Jennie, Thomas M. S. Wolever, M.D., Kaye Foster-Powell, and Stephen Colagiuri, M.D. *The Glycemic Revolution*. New York: Marlowe & Co. 1996, 1998, 1999, 2002, 2003.

Brownstein, Arlen, and Donna Schoemaker. *Rosacea: Your Self-Help Guide*. Oakland, Calif.: New Harbinger Publishing, 2001.

The Burton Goldberg Group. *Alternative Medicine: The Definitive Guide*. Tiburon, Calif.: Future Medicine Publishing, Inc., 1999.

Cherniske, Stephen. *Caffeine Blues*. New York: Warner Books, 1998.

Colbin, Annemarie. *Food and Healing*. New York: Ballantine Books, 1996.

Crook, William G. *The Yeast Connection: A Medical Breakthrough*. New York: Vintage Books, 1996.

Diamond, John W., M.D., and W. Lee Cowden, M.D., eds. *The Definitive Guide to Cancer*. Tiburon, Calif.: Future Medicine Publishing, Inc., 1997.

Duke, James A. *The Green Pharmacy: The Ultimate Compendium of Natural Remedies from the World's Foremost Authority on Healing Herbs*. Emmaus, Pa.: Rodale Press, 1997.

Epstein, Samuel, and David Steinman. *The Breast Cancer Prevention Program*. New York: Macmillan, 1997.

Epstein, Samuel, et al. *The Politics of Cancer Revisited*. Fremont Center, N.Y.: East Ridge Press, 1998.

Erasmus, Udo. *Fats That Heal, Fats That Kill: The Complete Guide to Fats, Oils, Cholesterol, and Human Health*. Burnaby, B.C., Canada: Alive Books, 1993.

Erickson, Kim. *Drop Dead Gorgeous*. Chicago: Contemporary Books, 2002.

Garcia, Oz. *Look and Feel Fabulous Forever*. New York: ReganBooks, 2002.

Gittleman, Ann Louise. *The Complete Fat Flush Program*. New York: McGraw-Hill/Contemporary Books, 2002.

Glenmullen, Joseph. *Prozac Backlash*. New York: Touchstone Books, 2001.

Hampton, Aubrey. *What's in Your Cosmetics? A Complete Consumer's Guide to Natural and Synthetic Ingredients*. Tuscon, Ariz.: Odonian Press, 1995.

Hampton, Aubrey, and Susan Hussey. *The Take Charge Beauty Book: The Ultimate Guide to Beautiful Hair and Skin*. Tampa, Fla.: Organica Press, 1999.

Jeffers, Susan. *Feel the Fear and Do it Anyway*. San Diego: Harcourt Brace Jovanovich, 1987.

Lark, Susan M., and James A. Richards. *The Chemistry of Success: Six Secrets of Peak Performance*. San Francisco, Calif.: Bay Books, 2000.

Larson, Joan Matthews. *Seven Weeks to Sobriety*. New York: Fawcett Books, 1997.

Lee, John R., with Virginia Hopkins. *What Your Doctor May Not Tell You About Menopause*. New York: Warner Books, 1996.

Lininger, Skye, D.C. (editor-in-chief), Alan Gaby, M.D., Steve Austin, N.D., Donald J. Brown, N.D., Forrest Batz, PharmD, and Eric Yarnell, N.D. *The A-Z Guide to Drug-Herb-Vitamin Interactions*. Rocklin, Calif.: Prima Health, 1999.

Lininger, Skye, D.C. (editor-in-chief), Alan Gaby, M.D., Steve Austin, N.D., Donald J. Brown, N.D., Jonathan V. Wright, M.D., and Alice Duncan, D.C., CCH. *The Natural Pharmacy*, 2nd ed. Rocklin, Calif.: Prima Health, 1999.

Medical Economics Staff. *PDR for Herbal Medicines*, 2nd ed. Montvale, N.J.: Medical Economics Company, 2000.

Murray, Michael T. *Natural Alternatives to Over-the-Counter and Prescription Drugs*. New York: Quill Books, 1999.

Northrup, Christiane. *The Wisdom of Menopause: Creating Physical and Emotional Health and Healing During the Change*. New York: Bantam Books, 2001.

Null, Gary. *Get Healthy Now! A Complete Guide to Prevention, Treatment, and Healthy Living*. New York: Seven Stories Press, 1999.

Perricone, Nicholas, M.D. *The Perricone Prescription*. New York: HarperCollins, 2002.

Pilzer, Paul. *The Wellness Revolution: How to Make a Fortune in the Next Trillion Dollar Industry*. New York: Wiley & Sons, 2002.

Raichur, Pratima, and Marian Raichur Cohn. *Absolute Beauty: Radiant Skin and Inner Harmony through the Ancient Secrets of Ayurveda*. New York: HarperCollins, 1997.

Reaven, Gerald M., Terry Kristen Strom, and Barry Fox. *Syndrome X, the Silent Killer: The New Heart Disease Risk*. New York: Fireside Books, 2001.

Rivera, Rudy, and Roger D. Deutsch. *Your Hidden Food Allergies Are Making You Fat: The ALCAT Food Sensitivities Weight Loss Breakthrough*, 2nd ed. Roseville, Calif.: Prima Publishing, 2002.

Rubin, Jordan S., N.M.D., C.N.C. *Patient, Heal Thyself*. Topanga, Calif.: Freedom Press, 2003.

Sears, Barry, and Bill Lawren. *The Zone: A Dietary Road Map to Lose Weight Permanently, Reset Your Genetic Code, Prevent Disease, Achieve Maximum Physical Performance*. New York: Regan Books, 1995.

Segala, Melanie, ed. *Disease Prevention and Treatment*, 4th ed. Fort Lauderdale, Fla.: Life Extension Foundation, 2003..

Steinman, David, and Samuel Epstein. *The Safe Shopper's Bible: A Consumer's Guide to Non-Toxic Household Products, Cosmetics, and Food*. New York: Macmillan USA, 1995.

Steinman, David, and R. Michael Wisner. *Living Healthy in a Toxic World: Simple Steps to Protect You and Your Family from Everyday Chemicals, Poisons, and Pollution*. New York: Berkley Publishing Group, 1996.

Vance, Judi. *Beauty to Die For*. San Jose, Calif.: To Excel, 1999.

Vanderhaeghe, Lorna R. *Healthy Immunity*. New York: Kensington Publishing Corp., 2001.

Wetherall, Charles F. *Quit: Read This Book and Stop Smoking*. Philadelphia, Pa.: Running Press, 2001.

Winter, Ruth. *A Consumers Dictionary of Cosmetic Ingredients*, 5th ed. New York: Three Rivers Press, 1999.

bibliography

Chapter 3

Adler, S. R., and J. R. Fosket. "Disclosing Complementary and Alternative Medicine Use in the Medical Encounter: A Qualitative Study in Women with Breast Cancer." *Journal of Family Practice* 48, no. 6 (June 1999): 453–58.

Adlercreutz, H., Y. Mousavi, J. Clark, K. Hockerstedt, E. Hamalainen, K. Wahala, T. Makela, and T. Hase. "Dietary Phytoestrogens and Cancer: In Vitro and In Vivo Studies." *Journal of Steroid Biochemistry and Molecular Biology* 41, no. 3–8 (March 1992): 331–37.

Arliss, R. M., and C. A. Biermann. "Do Soy Isoflavones Lower Cholesterol, Inhibit Atherosclerosis, and Play a Role in Cancer Prevention?" *Holistic Nursing Practice* 16, no. 5 (October 2002): 40–48.

Associated Press. "Canada Rejects P&G's Olestra." *Cincinnati Post*, 23 June 2000.

Challem, Jack. "Natural vs. Synthetic Vitamin E." *Nutrition Science News*, November 2001.

Cover, C. M., et al. "Indole-3-carbinol and Tamoxifen Cooperate to Arrest the Cell Cycle of MCF-7 Human Breast Cancer Cells." *Cancer Research* 59 (1999): 1244–51.

De Pinieux, G., P. Chariot, M. Ammi-Said, F. Louarn, J. L. Lejonc, A. Astier, B. Jacotot, and R. Gherardi. "Lipid-lowering Drugs and Mitochondrial Function: Effects of HMG-CoA Reductase Inhibitors on Serum Ubiquinone and Blood Lactate/

Pyruvate Ratio." *British Journal of Clinical Pharmacology* 42, no. 3 (September 1996): 333–37.

Erasmus, Udo. *Fats That Heal, Fats That Kill.* Burnaby, B.C., Canada: Alive Books, 1983, 1993.

Erickson, Kim. *Drop Dead Gorgeous.* New York, N.Y.: Contemporary Books, 2002.

"FDA: Authority over Cosmetics." U.S. Food and Drug Administration Center for Food Safety and Applied Nutrition, Office of Cosmetics and Colors, 3 February 1995.

Grady, Denise. "Risks of Hormone Therapy Exceed Benefits, Panel Says." *New York Times*, 17 October 2002.

Harding, Ann. "Broccoli-derived Pill May Help Ward Off Cancer." *Reuters Health*, 19 August 2002.

Hilts, Philip J. "U.S. Weighs Rule Changes on Conflicts in Drug Study." *New York Times*, 16 August 2000.

Horwitz, Ralph I., M.D., Lawrence M. Brass, M.D., Walter N. Kernan, M.D., and Catherine M. Viscoli, Ph.D. "Phenylpropanolamine and Risk of Hemorrhagic Stroke: Final Report of the Hemorrhagic Stroke Project." FDA submission, 10 May 2000.

Kolpin, Dana W., et al. "Pharmaceuticals, Hormones, and Other Organic Wastewater Contaminants in U.S. Streams, 1999–2000: A National Reconnaissance." *Environmental Science and Technology* 36 (2002): 1202–11.

Linde, K., et al. "St. John's Wort for Depression—an Overview and Meta-analysis of Randomised Clinical Trials." *British Medical Journal* 313, no. 7052 (3 August 1996): 253–58.

Morrow, Michele G., D.O. "A Celebration of First Amendment Victories Against the FDA." *Life Extension Magazine*, April 2002, p. 27.

Mulvihill, Keith. "Tobacco Company Influenced Nicotine Gum, Patch Ads." *Reuters Health*, 14 August 2002.

Pear, Robert. "Drug Industry Is Told to Stop Gifts to Doctors." *New York Times*, 1 October 2002.

Peterson, Melody. "Heartfelt Advice, Hefty Fees." *New York Times*, 11 August 2002.

Poole, K. "Mechanisms of Bacterial Biocide and Antibiotic Resistance." *Journal of Applied Microbiology* 92, supplement (2002): 55S–64S.

Pugh, Tony. "Doctors Are Sick of Drug Salesmen: Pharmaceutical Reps Face New Rules When Knocking on Doors." *Mercury News*, 2 September 2002.

Salaman, Maureen K., and Jonathan V. Wright. "Would You Buy a Used Car from FDA? Distorting the 'Pure Food' (and Other) Laws Since 1906." *Townsend Letter for Doctors* 133: 968–71.

Smeh, Nikolaus J. *Health Risks in Today's Cosmetics*. Garrison, Va.: Alliance Publishing, 1994, p. 14.

Stolberg, Sheryl Gay. "F.D.A. Ban Sought on Chemical Used for Cold Remedies." *New York Times*, 20 October 2000.

Taubes, Gary. "What If It's All Been a Big Fat Lie?" *New York Times*, 7 July 2002.

Uehling, Mark D. "Free Drugs from Your Faucet." *Salon* 25 (October 2002).

U.S. Preventive Services Task Force. "Postmenopausal Hormone Replacement Therapy for Primary Prevention of Chronic Conditions: Recommendations and Rationale." *Annals of Internal Medicine* 137 (2002): 834–39.

Vanderhaeghe, Lorna R. *Healthy Immunity*. New York: Twin Streams Books, 2001, p. 57.

Verrengia, Joseph B. "America's Waterways Contaminated by Medications, Personal Care Products." Associated Press, 13 March 2002. Environmental News Network Web site: *www.enn.com/news*

Warner, Jennifer. "Broccoli Pill Prevents Breast Cancer." *WebMD Medical News*, 19 August 2002.

Wong, N. C. "The Beneficial Effects of Plant Sterols on Serum Cholesterol." *Canadian Journal of Cardiology* 17, no. 6 (June 2001): 715–21.

Chapter 5

Aviram, M., L. Dornfeld, M. Rosenblat, et al. "Pomegranate Juice Consumption Reduces Oxidative Stress, Atherogenic Modifications to LDL, and Platelet Aggregation: Studies in Humans and in Atherosclerotic Apolipoprotein E-deficient Mice." *American Journal of Clinical Nutrition* 71 (2000): 1062–76.

Borghouts, L. B., and H. A. Keizer. "Exercise and Insulin Sensitivity: A Review." *International Journal of Sports Medicine* 21 (2000): 1–12 [review].

Cherniske, Stephen, M.S. *Caffeine Blues*. New York: Warner Books, 1998.

Curi R., M. Alvarez, R. B. Bazotte, et al. "Effect of Stevia Rebaudiana on Glucose Tolerance in Normal Adult Humans." *Brazilian Journal of Medical and Biological Research* 19 (1986): 771–74.

Dulloo, A. G., J. Sevdoux, L. Girardier, et al. "Green Tea and Thermogenesis: Interactions Between Catechin-polyphenols, Caffeine and Sympathetic Activity."

International Journal of Obesity and Related Metabolic Disorders 24, no. 2 (February 2000): 252–58.

Eliasson, B., S. Attvall, M. R. Taskinen, and U. Smith. "Smoking Cessation Improves Insulin Sensitivity in Healthy Middle-aged Men." *European Journal of Clinical Investigation* 27 (1997): 450–56.

Garland, E. M., and S. M. Cohen. "Saccharin-induced Bladder Cancer in Rats." *Progress in Clinical Biological Research* 391 (1995): 237–43 [review].

Geleijnse, J. M., L. J. Launer, D. A. Van der Kuip, A. Hofman, and J. C. Witteman. "Inverse Association of Tea and Flavonoid Intakes with Incident Myocardial Infarction: The Rotterdam Study." *American Journal of Clinical Nutrition* 75, no. 5 (May 2002): 880–86.

Hagino, N., and S. Ichimura. "Effects of Chlorella on Fecal and Urinary Cadmium Excretion in 'Itai-itai.'" *Japanese Journal of Hygiene* 30, no. 1 (1975): 77.

Hamajima, N., et al. "Alcohol, Tobacco and Breast Cancer—Collaborative Reanalysis of Individual Data from 53 Epidemiological Studies, including 58,515 Women with Breast Cancer and 95,067 Women without the Disease." *British Journal of Cancer* 87, no. 11 (18 November 2002): 1234–45.

Jakes, R. W., S. W. Duffy, F. C. Ng, F. Gao, E. H. Ng, A. Seow, H. P. Lee, and M. C. Yu. "Mammographic Parenchymal Patterns and Self-reported Soy Intake in Singapore Chinese Women." *Cancer Epidemiology, Biomarkers, and Prevention* 11, no. 7 (July 2002): 608–13.

Jenkins, D. J., M. Axelsen, C. W. Kendall, et al. "Dietary Fibre, Lente Carbohydrates and the Insulin-resistant Diseases." *British Journal of Nutrition* 83 (2000): S157–63 [review].

Katiyar, Santosh K., Mary S. Matsui, Craig A. Elmets, and Hasan Mukhtar. "Polyphenolic Antioxidant (-)-epigallocatechin-3-gallate from Green Tea Reduces UVB-inflammatory Responses and Infiltration of Leukocytes in Human Skin." *Photochemistry and Photobiology* 69, no. 2 (February 1999): 148–53.

Keijzers, G. B., B. E. De Galan, C. J. Tack, P. Smits. "Caffeine Can Decrease Insulin Sensitivity in Humans." *Diabetes Care* 25, no. 2 (February 2002): 364–69.

Kozlovsky, A., et al. "Effects of Diets High in Simple Sugars on Urinary Chromium Losses." *Metabolism* 35 (June 1986): 515–18.

Lark, Susan M., M.D., and James A. Richards, MBA. *The Chemistry of Success—Six Secrets of Peak Performance*. San Francisco: Bay Books, 2000.

Leung, A. Y., and S. Foster. *Encyclopedia of Common Natural Ingredients Used in Foods, Drugs, and Cosmetics*, 2nd ed. New York: John Wiley & Sons, 1996, pp. 478–80.

Lingelbach, L. B., A. E. Mitchell, R. B. Rucker, and R. B. McDonald. "Accumulation of Advanced Glycation Endproducts in Aging Male Fischer 344 Rats during Long-term Feeding of Various Dietary Carbohydrates." *Journal of Nutrition* 130, no. 5 (May 2000): 1247–55.

Nakachi, K., K. Suemasu, K. Suga, T. Takeo, K. Imai, and Y. Higashi. "Influence of Drinking Green Tea on Breast Cancer Malignancy among Japanese Patients." *Japanese Journal of Cancer Research* 89, no. 3 (1998): 254–61.

Ooshima, T., T. Minami, W. Aono, et al. "Reduction of Dental Plaque Deposition in Humans by Oolong Tea Extract." *Caries Research* 28 (1994): 146–49.

Pawlak, D. B., J. M. Bryson, G. S. Denyer, and J. C. Brand-Miller. "High Glycemic Index Starch Promotes Hypersecretion of Insulin and Higher Body Fat in Rats without Affecting Insulin Sensitivity." *Journal of Nutrition* 131, no. 1 (January 2001): 99–104.

Perricone, Nicholas, M.D. *The Perricone Prescription*. New York: HarperCollins, 2002.

Sasazuki, S., H. Komdama, K. Yoshimasu, et al. "Relation between Green Tea Consumption and Severity of Coronary Atherosclerosis among Japanese Men and Women." *Annals of Epidemiology* 10 (2000): 401–8.

Smith-Warner, S. A., D. Spiegelman, S. S. Yaun, P. A. van den Brandt, A. R. Folsom, R. A. Goldbohm, S. Graham, L. Holmberg, G. R. Howe, J. R. Marshall, A. B. Miller, J. D. Potter, F. E. Speizer, W. C. Willett, A. Wolk, and D. J. Hunter. "Alcohol and Breast Cancer in Women: A Pooled Analysis of Cohort Studies." *Journal of the American Medical Association* 279, no. 7 (18 February 1998): 535–40.

Stellman, S., and L. Garfinkel. "Short Report: Artificial Sweetener Use and Weight Changes among Women." *Preventive Medicine* 15 (1986): 195–202.

Uehara, M., J. Sugiura, and K. Sakurai. "A Trial of Oolong Tea in the Management of Recalcitrant Atopic Dermatitis." *Archives of Dermatology* 137 (2001): 42–43.

U.S. Food and Drug Administration. "Final Rule" for Sucralose, 21 CFR Part 172, Docket No. 87F-0086.

Warner, Jennifer. "Broccoli Pill Prevents Breast Cancer." *WebMD Medical News*, 19 August 2002.

White, J. R., Jr., J. Kramer, R. K. Campbell, and R. Bernstein. "Oral Use of a Topical Preparation Containing an Extract of Stevia Rebaudiana and the Chrysanthemum Flower in the Management of Hyperglycemia." *Diabetes Care* 17 (1994): 940.

Wilkison, W., K. H. Golding, P. K. Robinson, et al. "Mercury Removed by Immobilized Algae in Batch Culture Systems." *Journal of Applied Phycology* 2 (1990): 223–30.

Wolever, T. M. "Dietary Carbohydrates and Insulin Action in Humans." *British Journal of Nutrition* 83 (2000): S97–102 [review].

Woods, D. "U.S. Scientists Challenge Approval of Sweetener." *British Medical Journal* 313, no. 7054 (17 August 1996): 386.

Wu, C. H., Y. C. Yang, W. J. Yao, F. H. Lu, J. S. Wu, and C. J. Chang. "Epidemiological Evidence of Increased Bone Mineral Density in Habitual Tea Drinkers." *Archives of Internal Medicine* 162, no. 9 (13 May 2002): 1001–6.

Zaizen, Y., et al. "Antitumor Effects of Soybean Hypocotyls and Soybeans on the Mammary Tumor Induction by N-methyl-n-nitrosourea in F344 Rats." *Anticancer Research* 20, no. 3A (2000): 1439–44.

Chapter 6

Aga, M., K. Iwaki, Y. Ueda, S. Ushio, N. Masaki, S. Fukuda, T. Kimoto, M. Ikeda, and M. Kurimoto. "Preventive Effect of Coriandrum Sativum (Chinese Parsley) on Localized Lead Deposition in ICR Mice." *Journal of Ethnopharmacology* 77 (2001): 203–8.

Agarwal, K. C. "Therapeutic Actions of Garlic Constituents." *Medicinal Research Reviews* 16 (1996): 111–24.

Ammon, H. P., et al. "Mechanism of Anti-inflammatory Actions of Curcumin and Boswellic Acids." *Journal of Ethnopharmacology* 38 (1993): 113.

Atkins, Robert C., M.D. *Dr. Atkins' New Diet Revolution.* New York: HarperCollins, 2002.

"Barbequer Beware." *Life Extension Magazine,* November 2000.

Benbrook, Charles. "Evidence of the Magnitude and Consequences of the Roundup Ready Soybean Yield Drag from University-Based Varietal Trials in 1998." Ag BioTech InfoNet Technical Paper Number 1, 13 July 1999.

Berkson, D. Lindsey. *Hormone Deception.* Lincolnwood, Ill.: Contemporary Books, 2000.

Berrio, L. F., M. M. Polansky, and R. A. Anderson. "Insulin Activity: Stimulatory Effects of Cinnamon and Brewer's Yeast as Influenced by Albumin." *Hormone Research* 37 (1992): 225–29.

Birnbaum, L. "Addition of Conjugated Linoleic Acid to a Herbal Anticellulite Pill." *Advances in Therapy* 18, no. 5 (September–October 2001): 225–29.

Blaylock, Russell L., M.D. *Excitotoxins: The Taste That Kills.* Santa Fe, N.M.: Health Press, 1997.

Booth, Sarah L. "Vitamin K: Another Reason to Eat Your Greens." *Agricultural Research Magazine* 48, no. 1 (January 2000): 16–17.

Brignall, Matt. "Are Some Plant Foods More Health-Promoting than Others?" *Healthnotes Newswire*, 14 March 2002.

Chang, S. T., P. F. Chen, and S. C. Chang. "Antibacterial Activity of Leaf Essential Oils and Their Constituents from Cinnamomum Osmophloeum" *Journal of Ethnopharmacology* 77 (2001): 123–27.

"Cinnamon Extracts Boost Insulin Sensitivity." *Agricultural Research* 48 (2000): 21.

Ciolino, H. P., et al. "Effect of Curcumin on the Aryl Hydrocarbon Receptor and Cytochrome p450 1A1 in MCF-7 Human Breast Carcinoma Cells." *Biochemical Pharmacology* 56 (1998): 197–206.

Dashwood, R. H., et al. "Cancer Chemopreventive Mechanisms of Tea against Heterocyclic Amine Mutagens from Cooked Meat." *Proceedings of the Society for Experimental Biology and Medicine* 220 (1999): 239–43.

Dhiman, T. R., et al. "Conjugated Linoleic Acid Content of Milk from Cows Fed Different Diets." *Journal of Dairy Science* 82, no. 10 (October 1999): 2146–56.

Diamond, W. John, M.D., and W. Lee Cowden, M.D., with Burton Goldberg. *An Alternative Medicine Definitive Guide to Cancer.* Tiburon, Calif.: Future Medicine Publishing, 1997, p. 869.

Efendy, J. L., D. L. Simmons, G. R. Campbell, and J. H. Campbell. "The Effect of the Aged Garlic Extract, 'Kyolic', on the Development of Experimental Atherosclerosis." *Atherosclerosis* 132 (1997): 37–42.

Environmental Protection Agency. "National Sewage Sludge Survey: Availability of Information and Data, and Anticipated Impacts on Proposed Regulation." 40 CFR Part 503 (FRL-3857-2). *Federal Register* 55, no. 218 (9 November 1990): 47210.

Erasmus, Udo. *Fats That Heal, Fats That Kill.* Burnaby, B.C., Canada: Alive Books, 1993.

Ernst, E. "Cardioprotection and Garlic." *Lancet* 349 (1997): 131.

Friedman, M., ed. *Nutritional and Toxicological Consequences of Food Processing.* New York: Plenum Press, 1991.

Gaby, Alan R., M.D. "Eat Nuts for a Healthy Heart." *Healthnotes Newswire,* 1 August 2002.

Gijsbers, B. L., K. S. Jie, and C. Vermeer. "Effect of Food Composition on Vitamin K Absorption in Human Volunteers." *British Journal of Nutrition* 76, no. 2 (August 1996): 223–29.

Gilbert, Susan. "Fears Over Milk, Long Dismissed, Still Simmer." *New York Times,* 19 January 1999.

Glinsmann, W., H. Irausquin, and K. Youngmee. "Evaluation of Health Aspects of Sugar Contained in Carbohydrate Sweeteners." FDA Report of Sugars Task Force 39 (1986): 36–38.

"GM Crop DNA Found in Human Gut Bugs." *NewScientist.com* 12:10, 18 July 2002.

Guh, J. H., et al. "Antiplatelet Effect of Gingerol Isolated from Zingiber officinale." *Journal of Pharmacy and Pharmacology* 47 (1995): 329–32.

Healthnotes, Inc. "Cayenne as an herbal remedy." 2002. *www.mycostompak.com/healthnotes/herb/cayenne.htm*

Hidaka, H., T. Ishiko, T. Furuhashi, H. Kamohara, S. Suzuki, M. Miyazaki, et al. "Curcumin Inhibits Interleukin 8 Production and Enhances Interleukin 8 Receptor Expression on the Cell Surface: Impact on Human Pancreatic Carcinoma Cell Growth by Autocrine Regulation." *Cancer* 95 (2002): 1206–14.

Holtmann, S., A. H. Clarke, H. Scherer, and M. Hohn. "The Anti-motion Sickness Mechanism of Ginger: A Comparative Study with Placebo and Dimenhydrinate." *Acta Otolaryngologica* (Stockholm) 108 (1989): 168–74.

Horowitz, B. J., S. Edelstein, and L. Lippman. "Sugar Chromatography Studies in Recurrent Candida Vulvovaginitis." *Journal of Reproductive Medicine* 29 (1984): 441–43.

Jenkins, D. J., C. W. Kendall, A. Marchie, T. L. Parker, P. W. Connelly, W. Qian, J. S. Haight, D. Faulkner, E. Vidgen, K. G. Lapsley, and G. A. Spiller. "Dose Response of Almonds on Coronary Heart Disease Risk Factors: Blood Lipids, Oxidized Low-density Lipoproteins, Lipoprotein(a), Homocysteine, and Pulmonary Nitric Oxide: A Randomized, Controlled, Crossover Crial." *Circulation* 106, no. 11 (10 September 2002): 1327–32.

Kekwick, A., and G. L. S. Pawan. "Calorie Intake in the Relation to Body Weight Changes in the Obese." *Lancet* 2 (1956): 155–61.

Kiso, Y., Y. Suzuki, N. Watanbe, et al. "Antihepatotoxic Principles of Curcuma longa Rhizomes." *Planta Medica* 49 (1983): 185–87.

Kozlovsky, A., et al. "Effects of Diets High in Simple Sugars on Urinary Chromium Losses." *Metabolism* 35 (1986): 515–18.

Lark, Susan M. "My Philosophy on Weight Loss and Management." *The Lark Letter* 9, no. 2 (February 2002) (Phillips Health, LLC, Potomac, Maryland).

Lee, A. T., and A. Cerami. "The Role of Glycation in Aging." *Annals of the New York Academy of Science* 663 (1992): 63–70.

Lingelbach, L. B., A. E. Mitchell, R. B. Rucker, and R. B. McDonald. "Accumulation of Advanced Glycation Endproducts in Aging Male Fischer 344 Rats during Long-term Feeding of Various Dietary Carbohydrates." *Journal of Nutrition* 130, no. 5 (May 2000): 1247–55.

Mehta, K., et al. "Antiproliferative Effect of Curcumin (Diferuloylmethane) against Human Breast Tumor Cell Line." *Anticancer Drugs* 8 (1997): 470–81.

Mellon, Margaret, Charles Benbrook, and Karen Lutz Benbrook. "Hogging It: Estimates of Antimicrobial Abuse in Livestock." Cambridge, Mass.: Union of Concerned Scientists, 2001, p. xiii.

Mitchell, Terri. "A Report on Curcumin's Anti-cancer Effects." *Life Extension Magazine*, July 2002, pp. 27–30.

Mokdad, A. H., E. S. Ford, B. A. Bowman, et al. "Prevalence of Obesity, Diabetes, and Other Obesity-related Health Risk Factors, 2001." *Journal of the American Medical Association* 289, no. 1 (1 January 2003): 76–79.

Monnier, V. M. "Nonenzymatic Glycosylation, the Maillard Reaction and the Aging Process." *Journal of Gerontology* 454 (1990): 105–10.

Moschos, S. J., and C. S. Mantzoros. "The Role of the IGF System in Cancer: From Basic to Clinical Studies and Clinical Applications." *Oncology* 63, no. 4 (2002): 317–32 [review].

Nerurkar, P. V., et al. "Effects of Marinating with Asian Marinades or Western Barbecue Sauce on PhIP and MelQx Formation in Barbecued Beef." *Nutrition and Cancer* 34 (1999): 147–52.

Organic Consumers Association Web site: *www.organicconsumers.org*

Pariza, M. W., Y. Park, and M. E. Cook. "Conjugated Linoleic Acid and the Control of Cancer and Obesity." *Toxicological Sciences* 52, supplement 2 (December 1999): 107–10.

Pawlak, D. B., J. M. Bryson, G. S. Denyer, and J. C. Brand-Miller. "High Glycemic Index Starch Promotes Hypersecretion of Insulin and Higher Body Fat in Rats without Affecting Insulin Sensitivity." *Journal of Nutrition* 131, no. 1 (January 2001): 99–104.

Perricone, Nicholas, M.D. *The Perricone Prescription*. New York: HarperCollins, 2002, p. 34.

Phillips, S., et al. "Zingiber Officinale (Ginger)—An Antiemetic for Day Case Surgery." *Anaesthesia* 48 (1993): 715–17.

Prineas, R. J., G. Grandits, P. M. Rautaharju, J. D. Cohen, Z. M. Zhang, and R. S. Crow. "Long-term Prognostic Significance of Isolated Minor Electrocardiographic T-wave Abnormalities in Middle-aged Men Free of Clinical Cardiovascular Disease (The Multiple Risk Factor Intervention Trial [MRFIT])." *American Journal of Cardiology* 90 (2002): 1391–95.

Ruby, A. J., et al. "Anti-tumour and Antioxidant Activity of Natural Curcuminoids." *Cancer Letters* 94 (1995): 79–83.

Sanchez, A., et al. "Role of Sugars in Human Neutrophilic Phagocytosis." *American Journal of Clinical Nutrition* 261 (1973): 1180–84.

Scanto, S., and J. Yudkin. "The Effect of Dietary Sucrose on Blood Lipids, Serum Insulin, Platelet Adhesiveness and Body Weight in Human Volunteers." *Postgraduate Medicine Journal* 45 (1969): 602–7.

Sears, Barry, Ph.D. *The Zone*. New York: ReganBooks, 1995, p. 21.

Spears, Tom. "GE Canola Superweeds Spread Across Canada." *The Ottawa Citizen*, 6 February 2001.

Steiner, M., et al. "A Double-blind Crossover Study in Moderately Hypercholesterolemic Men that Compared the Effect of Aged Garlic Extract and Placebo Administration on Blood Lipids." *American Journal of Clinical Nutrition* 64 (1996): 866–70.

Suekawa, M., et al. "Pharmacological Studies on Ginger, I. Pharmacological Actions of Pungent Constitutents, (6)-gingerol and (6)-shogaol." *Journal of Pharmacobio-Dynamics* 7 (1984): 836–48.

Thomas, B. J., R. J. Jarrett, H. Keen, and H. J. Ruskin. "Relation of Habitual Diet to Fasting Plasma Insulin Concentration and the Insulin Response to Oral Glucose." *Human Nutrition Clinical Nutrition* 36C, no. 1 (1982): 49–56.

Vutyavanich, T., T. Kraisarin, and R. Ruangsri. "Ginger for Nausea and Vomiting in Pregnancy: Randomized, Double-masked, Placebo-controlled Trial." *Obstetrics and Gynecology* 97 (2001): 577–82.

Yamahara, J, et al. "Cholagogic Effect of Ginger and Its Active Constituents." *Journal of Ethnopharmacology* 13 (1985): 217.

Yamahara, J., H. Q. Rong, Y. Naitoh, et al. "Inhibition of Cytotoxic Drug-induced Vomiting in Suncus by a Ginger Constituent." *Journal of Ethnopharmacology* 27 (1989): 353–55.

Zambon, D., J. Sabate, S. Munoz, B. Campero, E. Casals, M. Merlos, J. C. Laguna, and E. Ros. "Substituting Walnuts for Monounsaturated Fat Improves the Serum Lipid Profile of Hypercholesterolemic Men and Women: A Randomized Crossover Trial." *Annals of Internal Medicine* 132, no. 7 (2000): 538–46.

Chapter 7

Bernstein, J., et al. "Depression of Lymphosyte Transformation Following Oral Glucose Ingestion." *American Journal of Clinical Nutrition* 30 (1997): 613.

Persson, P., A. Ahlbom, and G. Hellers. "Diet and Inflammatory Bowel Disease: A Case-Control Study." *Epidemiology* 3, no. 1 (January 1992): 47–52.

Chapter 8

Anand, I., Y. Chandrashenkhan, F. De Giuli, et al. "Acute and Chronic Effect of Propionyl-L-carnitine on the Hemodynamics, Exercise Capacity and Hormones of Patients with Congestive Heart Failure." *Cardiovascular Drugs and Therapy* 12 (1998): 291–99.

Anderson, R. A. "Chromium, Glucose Intolerance and Diabetes." *Journal of the American College of Nutrition* 17 (1998): 548–55.

Anderson, R. A., et al. "Elevated Intakes of Supplemental Chromium Improve Glucose and Insulin Variables in Individuals with Type 2 Diabetes." *Diabetes* 46, no. 11 (November 1997): 1786–91.

Balz, F. "Antioxidant Vitamins and Heart Disease." Paper presented at the 60th Annual Biology Colloquium, Oregon State University, Corvallis, Oregon, 25 February 1999.

Baskaran, K., et al. "Antidiabetic Effect of a Leaf Extract from Gymnema Sylvestre in Non-insulin-dependent Diabetes Mellitus Patients." *Journal of Ethnopharmacology* 30, no. 3 (October 1990): 295–300.

Bjørneboe, A., E. Søyland, G. E. Bjørneboe, et al. "Effect of Dietary Supplementation with Eicosapentaenoic Acid in the Treatment of Atopic Dermatitis." *British Journal of Dermatology* 117 (1987): 463–69.

Bjørneboe, A., E. Søyland, G. E. Bjørneboe, et al. "Effect of n-3 Fatty Acid Supplement to Patients with Atopic Dermatitis." *Journal of Internal Medicine: Supplement* 225 (1989): 233–36.

Blask, D. E., L. A. Sauer, and R. T. Dauchy. "Melatonin as a Chronobiotic/Anticancer Agent: Cellular, Biochemical, and Molecular Mechanisms of Action and Their Implications for Circadian-based Cancer Therapy." *Current Topics in Medical Chemistry* 2, no. 2 (February 2002): 113–32 [review].

Boldyrev, A., R. Song, D. Lawrence, et al. "Carnosine Protects against Excitotoxic Cell Death Independently of Effects on Reactive Oxygen Species." *Neuroscience* 94 (1999): 571–77.

Boldyrev, A., S. L. Stvolinsky, O. V. Tyulina, et al. "Biochemical and Physiological Evidence that Carnosine Is an Endogenous Neuroprotector against Free Radicals." *Cellular and Molecular Neurobiology* 17, no. 2 (1997): 259–71.

Brownson, C., and A. R. Hipkiss. "Carnosine Reacts with a Glycated Protein." *Free Radical Biology and Medicine* 28, no. 10 (2000): 1564–70.

Calder, P. C., and S. Kew. "The Immune System: A Target for Functional Foods?" *British Journal of Nutrition* 88, supplement 2 (2002): S165–77.

Caruso, I., et al. "Double-blind Study of 5http Versus Placebo in the Treatment of Primary Fibromyalgia Syndrome." *Journal of International Medical Research* 18 (May–June 1990): 201–9.

Ceconi, C., S. Curello, A. Cargnoni, et al. "The Role of Glutathione Status in the Protection against Ischaemic and Reperfusion Damage: Effects of N-acetyl cysteine." *Journal of Molecular and Cellular Cardiology* 20 (1988): 5–13.

Cheema-Dhadli, S., M. L. Harlperin, and C. C. Leznoff. "Inhibition of Enzymes which Interact with Citrate by (-)hydroxycitrate and 1,2,3,-tricarboxybenzene." *European Journal of Biochemistry* 38 (1973): 98–102.

Chernomorsky, S. A., and A. B. Segelman. "Biological Activities of Chlorophyll Derivatives." *New Jersey Medicine* 85 (1988): 669–73.

Chou, F. P., Y. D. Chu, J. D. Hsu, H. C. Chiang, and C. J. Wang. "Specific Induction of Glutathione S-transferase GSTM2 Subunit Expression by Epigallocatechin Gallate in Rat Liver." *Biochemical Pharmacology* 60, no. 5 (1 September 2000): 643–50.

Clark, L. C., G. F. Combs Jr., B. W. Turnbull, et al. "Effects of Selenium Supplementation for Cancer Prevention in Patients with Carcinoma of the Skin: A Randomized Controlled Trial." Nutritional Prevention of Cancer Study Group. *Journal of the American Medical Association* 276 (1996): 1957–63.

Cover, C. M., et al. "Indole-3-carbinol Inhibits the Expression of Cyclin-dependent Kinase-6 and Induces a G1 Cell Cycle Arrest of Human Breast Cancer Cells Independent of Estrogen Receptor Signaling." *Journal of Biological Chemistry* 273 (1998): 3838–47.

Curley, R. W., Jr., et al. "Activity of D-glucarate Analogues: Synergistic Antiproliferative Effects with Retinoid in Cultured Human Mammary Tumor Cells Appear to Specifically Require the D-glucarate Structure." *Life Sciences* 54, no. 18 (1994): 1299–1303.

Diamond, W. John, M.D., and W. Lee Cowden, M.D., with Burton Goldberg. *An Alternative Medicine Definitive Guide to Cancer.* Tiberon, Calif.: Future Medicine Publishing, 1997, p. 570.

Diehm, C., H. J. Trampisch, S. Lange, and C. Schmidt. "Comparison of Leg Compression Stocking and Oral Horse-chestnut Seed Extract Therapy in Patients with Chronic Venous Insufficiency." *Lancet* 347, no. 8997 (1996): 292–94.

Diehm, C., D. Vollbrecht, K. Amendt, and H. U. Comberg. "Medical Edema Protection—Clinical Benefit in Patients with Chronic Deep Vein Incompetence: A Placebo-controll Double-blind Study." *Vasa* 21, no. 2 (1992): 188–92.

Digiesi, V., R. Palchetti, and F. Cantini. "The Benefits of L-carnitine in Essential Arterial Hypertension." *Minerva Medica* 80 (1989): 227–31.

Dulloo, A. G., C. Duret, D. Rohrer, L. Girardier, N. Mensi, M. Fathi, P. Chantre, and J. Vandermander. "Efficacy of a Green Tea Extract Rich in Catechin Polyphenols and Caffeine in Increasing 24-h Energy Expenditure and Fat Oxidation in Humans." *American Journal of Clinical Nutrition* 70, no. 6 (December 1999): 1040–45.

Fuchs, C. S., et al. "The Influence of Folate and Multivitamin Use on the Familial Risk of Colon Cancer in Women." *Cancer Epidemiology, Biomarkers, and Prevention* 11 (2002): 227–34.

Fuchs, Nan Catherine. "Q & A." *Women's Health Letter* 8 (January 1999), p. 8.

Fujita, T., Y. Fujii, B. Goto, A. Miyauchi, and Y. Takagi. "Peripheral Computed Tomography (pQCT) Detected Short-term Effect of AAACa (Heated Oyster Shell with Heated Algal Ingredient HAI): A Double-blind Comparison with CaCO3 and Placebo." *Journal of Bone and Mineral Metabolism* 18 (2000): 212–15.

Gaby, A. R. "The Role of Coenzyme Q10 in Clinical Medicine: Part II. Cardiovascular Disease, Hypertension, Diabetes Mellitus and Infertility." *Alternative Medicine Review* 1 (1996): 168–75.

Ganguli, S., et al. "Effects of Maternal Vanadate Treatment of Fetal Development." *Life Sciences* 55, no. 16 (1994): 1267–76.

Gruskin, B. "Chlorophyll—Its Therapeutic Place in Acute and Suppurative Disease." *American Journal of Surgery* 49 (1940): 49–56.

Guthrie, N., et al. "Inhibition of Proliferation of Estrogen Receptor-negative MDA-MB-435 and –positive MCF-7 Human Breast Cancer Cells by Palm Oil Tocotrienols and Tamoxifen, Alone and in Combination." *Journal of Nutrition* 127 (March 1997): 544S–48S.

Hagen, T. M., et al. "Acetyl-L-carnitine Fed to Old Rats Partially Restores Mitochondrial Function and Ambulatory Activity." *Proceedings of the National Academy of Sciences* 95, no. 16 (4 August 1998): 9562–66.

Hagen, T. M., et al. "Feeding Acetyl-L-carnitine and Lipoic Acid to Old Rats Significantly Improves Metabolic Function while Decreasing Oxidative Stress." *Proceedings of the National Academy of Sciences* 99, no. 4 (19 February 2002): 1870–75.

Hagen, T. M., C. M. Wehr, and B. N. Ames. "Mitochondrial Decay in Aging: Reversal through Supplementation of cetyl-L-carnitine and N-tertbutyl-alpha-phenylnitrone." *Annals of the New York Academy of Sciences* 854 (November 1998): 214–23.

Hagino, N., and S. Ichimura. "Effects of Chlorella on Fecal and Urinary Cadmium Excretion in 'Itai-itai.'" *Japanese Journal of Hygiene* 30, no. 1 (1975): 77.

Hayatsu, H., T. Negishi, S. Arimoto, et al. "Porphyrins as Potential Inhibitors against Exposure to Carcinogens and Mutagens." *Mutation Research* 290 (1993): 79–85.

Heerdt, A. S., et al. "Calcium Glucarate as a Chemopreventive Agent in Breast Cancer." *Journal of Medical Sciences* (Israel) 31, nos. 2–3 (1995): 101–5.

Hibbeln, J. R., et al. "Dietary Polyunsaturated Fatty Acids and Depression: When Cholesterol Does Not Satisfy." *American Journal of Clinical Nutrition* 62 (1995): 1–9.

Hoeger, W. W., C. Harris, E. M. Long, and D. R. Hopkins. "Four-week Supplementation with a Natural Dietary Compound Produces Favorable Changes in Body

Composition." *Advances in Therapy* 15, no. 5 (September–October 1998): 305–14.

Holtzman, David. "All in the Genes." *Life Extension Magazine*, March 2001, p. 23.

Hoover, R. N. "Cancer—Nature, Nurture or Both?" *New England Journal of Medicine* 343 (13 July 2000): 135–36.

Horrobin, D. "Essential Fatty Acids in Clinical Dermatology." *Journal of the American Academy of Dermatology* 20 (June 1989): 1045–53.

Horrobin, D. "How Do Polyunsaturated Fatty Acids Lower Plasma Cholesterol Levels?" *Lipids* 18, no. 8 (August 1983): 558–62.

Horrobin, D. F. "The Importance of Gamma-linolenic Acid and Prostaglandin E1 in Human Nutrition and Medicine." *Journal of Holistic Medicine* 3 (1981): 118–39.

Ingels, Darin. "Diglyceride-Rich Foods May Promote Weight Loss." *Healthnotes Newswire*, 23 January 2003.

Isseroff, R. R. "Fish Again for Dinner! The Role of Fish and Other Dietary Oils in the Therapy of Skin Disease." *Journal of the American Academy of Dermatology* 19 (December 1988): 1073–80.

Iwamoto, J., T. Takeda, S. Ichimura, and M. Uzawa. "Effects of Five-year Treatment with Elcatonin and Alfacalcidol on Lumbar Bone Mineral Density and the Incidence of Vertebral Fractures in Postmenopausal Women with Osteoporosis: A Retrospective Study." *Journal of Orthopaedic Science* 7 (2002): 637–43.

Jacob, S., et al. "Enhancement of Glucose Disposal in Patients with Type 2 Diabetes by Alpha-lipoic Acid." *Arzneimittelforschung* 45, no. 8 (August 1995): 872–74.

Jordan, Karin G., M.D. "Can Silibinin Arrest Cancer Cells Growth?" *Life Extension Magazine*, June 2000, p. 27.

Jordan, Karin G., M.D. "Nature's Pluripotent Life Extension Agent." *Life Extension Magazine*, January 2001, p. 27.

Jovanovic-Peterson, L., M. Cutierrez, and C. M. Peterson. "Chromium Supplementation for Gestational Diabetic Women (DGM) Improves Glucose Tolerance and Decreases Hyperinsulinemia." *Diabetes* 45, supplement 2 (1996): 337A.

Kaats, G., K. Blum, J. Fisher, and J. Adelman. "Effects of Chromium Picolinate Supplementation on Body Composition: A Randomized, Double-masked, Placebo-controlled Study." *Current Therapeutic Research* 57 (1996): 747–56.

Kaats, G., K. Blum, D. Pullin, et al. "A Randomized, Double-masked, Placebo-controlled Study of the Effects of Chromium Picolinate Supplementation on

Body Composition: A Replication and Extension of a Previous Study." *Current Therapeutic Research* 59 (1998): 379–88.

Kagan, V., S. Khan, C. Swanson, et al. "Antioxidant Action of Thioctic Acid and Dihydrolipoic Acid." *Free Radical Biology and Medicine* 9S (1990): 15.

Katiyar, S. K., B. M. Bergamo, P. K. Vyalil, and C. A. Elmets. "Green Tea Polyphenols: DNA Photodamage and Photoimmunology." *Journal of Photochemistry and Photobiology B* 65 (2001): 109–14.

Khosraviani, K., et al. "Effect of Folate Supplementaion on Mucosal Cell Proliferation in High Risk Patients for Colon Cancer." *Gut* 51 (2002): 195–99.

Kramer, J. M. "N-3 Fatty Acid Supplements in Rheumatoid Arthritis." *American Journal of Clinical Nutrition* 71, supplement 1 (2000): 349S–51S.

Kuriyama, K., T. Shimizu, T. Horiguchi, M. Watabe, and Y. Abe. "Vitamin E Ointment at High Dose Levels Suppresses Contact Dermatitis in Rats by Stabilizing Keratinocytes." *Inflammation Research* 51, no. 10 (October 2002): 483–89.

Laird, R. D., and V. A. Drill. "Lipotropic Activity of Inositol and Chlortetracycline Alone and in Various Combinations of Choline, Vitamin B 12 and Folic Acid: Activity of Three Liver Extracts with Assays for These Substances." *Archives Internationales de Pharmacodynamie et de Therapie* 194, no. 1 (November 1971): 103–16.

Landi, G. "Oral Administration of Borage Oil in Atopic Dermatitis." *Journal of Applied Cosmetology* 11 (1993): 115–20.

Lau, C. S., et al. "Effects of Fish Oil Supplementation on Non-steroidal Anti-inflammatory Drug Requirement in Patients with Mild Rheumatoid Arthritis—A Double-blind Placebo Controlled Study. *British Journal of Rheumatology* 32 (1993): 982–89.

La Vecchia, C., E. Negri, C. Pelucchi, and S. Franceschi. "Dietary Folate and Colorectal Cancer." *International Journal of Cancer* 102, no. 5 (10 December 2002): 545–47.

Lefavi, R., R. Anderson, R. Keith, et al. "Efficacy of Chromium Supplementation in Athletes: Emphasis on Anabolism." *International Journal of Sport Nutrition* 2 (1992): 111–22.

Leventhal, L. J., et al. "Treatment of Rheumatoid Arthritis with Blackcurrant Seed Oil." *British Journal of Rheumatology* 33 (1994): 847–52.

Liu, J., et al. "Age-associated Mitochondrial Oxidative Decay: Improvement of Carnitine Acetyltranferase Substrate-binding Affinity and Activity in Brain by Feeding Old Rats Acetyl-L-carnitine and/or R-alpha-lipoic Acid." *Proceedings of the National Academy of Sciences* 99 (2002): 1876–81.

Liu, J., et al. "Memory Loss in Old Rats is Associated with Brain Mitochondrial Decay and RNA/DNA Oxidation: Partial Reversal by Feeding acetyl-L-carnitine and/or R-alpha-lipoic Acid." *Proceedings of the National Academy of Sciences* 99 (2002): 2356–61.

Lockwood, K., et al. "Progress on Therapy of Breast Cancer with Vitamin Q10 and the Regression of Metastases." *Biochemical and Biophysical Research Communications* 212 (1995): 172–77.

Majamaa, H. "Probiotics: A Novel Approach in the Management of Food Allergy." *Journal of Allergy and Clinical Immunology* 99, no. 2 (1997): 179–85.

Mancini, M., F. Rengo, M. Lingetti, et al. "Controlled Study on the Therapeutic Efficacy of Propionyl-L-carnitine in Patients with Congestive Heart Failure." *Arzneimittelforschung* 42 (1992): 1101–4.

McDonough, F. E., A. D. Hitchins, N. P. Wong, et al. "Modification of Sweet Acidophilus Milk to Improve Utilization by Lactose-intolerant Persons." *American Journal of Clinical Nutrition* 45 (1987): 570–74.

Mel'nikova, V. M., N. M. Gracheva, G. P. Belikov, et al. "The Chemoprophylaxis and Chemotherapy of Opportunistic Infections." *Antibiotiki i Khimioterapiia* 38 (1993): 44–48.

Mertz, W. "Chromium in Human Nutrition: A Review." *Journal of Nutrition* 123 (1993): 626–33.

Mischoulon, D., and M. Fava. "Docosahexanoic Acid and Omega-3 Fatty Acids in Depression." *Psychiatric Clinics of North America* 23 (2000): 785–94.

Mori, H., K. Niwa, Q. Zheng, Y. Yamada, K. Sakata, and N. Yoshimi. "Cell Proliferation in Cancer Prevention: Effects of Preventive Agents on Estrogen-related Endometrial Carcinogenesis Model and on an In Vitro Model in Human Colorectal Cells." *Mutation Research* 480–81 (1 September 2001): 201–7.

Mortensen, S. A., A. Leth, E. Agner, and M. Rohde. "Dose-related Decrease of Serum Coenzyme Q10 during Treatment with HMG-CoA Reductase Inhibitors." *Molecular Aspects of Medicine* 18, supplement (1997): S137–44.

Muzzarelli, R. A. "Clinical and Biochemical Evaluation of Chitosan for Hypercholesterolemia and Overweight Control." *Experientia Supplementa* (*EXS*) 87 (1999): 293–304.

Nakachi, K., K. Suemasu, K. Suga, T. Takeo, K. Imai, and Y. Higashi. "Influence of Drinking Green Tea on Breast Cancer Malignancy among Japanese Patients." *Japanese Journal of Cancer Research* 89, no. 3 (1998): 254–61.

"Natural News and Notes: Incredible Shrinking Nutrition." *Better Nutrition*, October 2002.

Nesaretnam, K., R. Stephen, R. Dils, and P. Darbre. "Tocotrienols Inhibit the Growth of Human Breast Cancer Cells Irrespective of Estrogen Receptor Status." *Lipids* 33 (1998): 461–69.

Newbene, P. M., K. M. Nauss, and J. L. de Camargo. "Lipotropes, Immunocompetence, and Cancer." *Cancer Research* 43, supplement 5 (May 1983): 2426S–34S.

Newberne. P. M. "Lipotropic Factors and Oncogenesis." *Advances in Experimental Medicine and Biology* 206 (1986): 223–51.

Nusgens, B. V., P. Humbert, A. Rougier, et al. "Stimulation of Collagen Biosynthesis by Topically Applied Vitamin C." *European Journal of Dermatology* 12 (2002): xxxii–xxxiv.

Oda, T. "Effect of Coenzyme Q10 on Stress-induced Cardiac Dysfunction in Paediatric Patients with Mitral Valve Prolapse: A Study by Stress Echocardiography." *Drugs under Experimental and Clinical Research* 11 (1985): 557–76.

Ohia, S. E., C. A. Opere, A. M. LeDay, et al. "Safety and Mechanism of Appetite Suppression by a Novel Hydroxycitric Acid Extract (HCA-SX)." *Molecular and Cellular Biochemistry* 238 (2002): 89–103.

Paradies, G., G. Petrosillo, M. N. Gadaleta, F. M. Ruggiero. "The Effect of Aging and Acetyl-L-carnitine on the Pyruvate Transport and Oxidation in Rat Heart Mitochondria." *FEBS [Federation of European Biochemical Societies] Letters* 454 (July 1999): 207–9.

Peet, M., and D. F. Horrobin. "A Dose-ranging Study of the Effects of Ethyl-eicosapentaenoate in Patients with Ongoing Depression Despite Apparently Adequate Treatment with Standard Drugs." *Archives of General Psychiatry* 59 (October 2002): 913–19.

Perricone, Nicholas, M.D. *The Perricone Prescription*. New York: HarperCollins, 2002, p. 129.

Picard, Andre. "Today's Fruits, Vegetables Lack Yesterday's Nutrition." *The Globe and Mail*, 6 July 2002.

Pinnell, S. R. "Cutaneous Photodamage, Oxidative Stress, and Topical Antioxidant Protection." *Journal of the American Academy of Dermatology* 48, no. 1 (January 2003): 1–19.

Pool-Zobel, B. L., A. Bub, H. Muller, I. Wollowski, and G. Rechkemmer. "Consumption of Vegetables Reduces Genetic Damage in Humans: First Results of a Human Intervention Trial with Carotenoid-rich Foods." *Carcinogenesis* 18 (1997): 1847–50.

Riales, R., and M. J. Albrink. "Effect of Chromium Chloride Supplementation on Glucose Tolerance and Serum Lipids including High-density Lipoprotein of Adult Men." *American Journal of Clinical Nutrition* 34 (1981): 2670–78.

Riserus, U., L. Berglund, and B. Vessby. "Conjugated Linoleic Acid (CLA) Reduced Abdominal Adipose Tissue in Obese Middle-aged Men with Signs of the Metabolic Syndrome: A Randomised Controlled Trial." *International Journal of Obesity and Related Metabolic Disorders* 25, no. 8 (August 2001): 1129–35.

Rohr, U. D., and J. Herold. "Melatonin Deficiencies in Women." *Maturitas* 41, supplement 1 (April 2002): S85–104.

Rose, D. P., and J. M. Conolley. "Omega-3 Fatty Acids as Cancer Chemopreventive Agents." *Pharmacology and Therapeutics* 83 (1999): 217–44.

Sajithlal, G. B., P. Chithra, and G. Chandrakasan. "Advanced Glycation End Products Induce Cross-linking of Collagen In Vitro." *Biochimica Biophysica Acta* 1407 (1998): 215–24.

Scambia, G., et al. "Antiproliferative Effect of Silybin on Gynaecological Malignancies: Synergism with Cisplatin and Doxorubicin." *European Journal of Cancer* 32A (1996): 877–82.

Schechter, Steven. "Fat Intake Can Boost Weight Loss, if We Are Selective about Our Choices." *Better Nutrition*, June 1997, p. 26.

Schellenberg, R. "Treatment for the Premenstrual Syndrome with Agnus Castus Fruit Extract: Prospective, Randomized, Placebo Controlled Study." *British Medical Journal* 20 (2001): 134–37.

Schernhammer, E. S., et al. "Rotating Night Shifts and Risk of Breast Cancer in Women Participating in the Nurses' Health Study." *Journal of the National Cancer Institute* 93 (17 October 2001): 1563–68.

Schlumpf, Margaret, Beata Cotton, Marianne Conscience, Vreni Haller, Beate Steinmann, and Walter Lichtensteiger. "In Vitro and In Vivo Estrogenicity of UV Screens." *Environmental Health Perspectives* 109 (March 2001): 239–44.

Schnyder, G., et al. "Decreased Rate of Coronary Restenosis after Lowering of Plasma Homocysteine Levels." *New England Journal of Medicine* 345 (2001): 1593–600.

Schonheit, K., L. Gille, and H. Nohl. "Effect of Alpha-lipoic Acid and Dihydrolipoic Acid on Ischemia/Reperfusion Injury of the Heart and Heart Mitochondria." *Biochimica Biophysica Acta* 9 (June 1995): 335–42.

Schrauzer, G. N., et al. "Cancer Mortality Correlation Studies—III: Statistical Associations with Dietary Selenium Intakes." *Bioinorganic Chemistry* 7 (1977): 23–31.

Shanmugasundaram, E. R., et al. "Use of Gymnema Sylvestre Leaf Extract in the Control of Blood Glucose in Insulin-dependent Diabetes Mellitus." *Journal of Ethnopharmacology* 30, no. 3 (October 1990): 281–94.

Shao, Z. M., Z. Z. Shen, C. H. Liu, M. R. Sartippour, V. L. Go, D. Heber, and M. Nguyen. "Curcumin Exerts Multiple Suppressive Effects on Human Breast Carcinoma Cells." *International Journal of Cancer* 98, no. 2 (10 March 2002): 234–40.

Singer, Sydney Ross, and Soma Grismaijer. *Dressed to Kill: The Link between Breast Cancer and Bras.* Pahoa, Hawaii: ISCD Press, 1995.

Smirnov, V. V., S. R. Reznik, V. A. V'iunitskaia, et al. "The Current Concepts of the Mechanisms of the Therapeutic-prophylactic Action of Probiotics from Bacteria in the Genus Bacillus." *Mikrobiolohichnyi Zhurnal* 55 (1993): 92–112.

Søyland, E., G. Rajka, A. Bjørneboe, et al. "The Effect of Eicosapentaenoic Acid in the Treatment of Atopic Dermatitis: A Clinical Study." *Acta Dermato-Venereologica* (Stockholm) 144, supplement (1989): 139.

St-Onge, M. P., C. Bourque, P. J. Jones, R. Ross, and W. E. Parsons. "Medium- versus Long-chain Triglycerides for Twenty-seven Days Increases Fat Oxidation and Energy Expenditure without Resulting in Changes in Body Composition in Overweight Women." *International Journal of Obesity and Related Metabolic Disorders* 27, no. 1 (January 2003): 95–102.

Suarna, C., R. L. Hood, R. T. Dean, and R. Stocker. "Comparative Antioxidant Activity of Tocotrienols and Other Natural Lipid-soluble Antioxidants in a Homogeneous System, and in Rat and Human Lipoproteins." *Biochimica Biophysica Acta* 1166 (1993): 163–70.

Sullivan, A. C., J. G. Hamilton, O. N. Miller, et al. "Inhibition of Lipogenesis in Rat Liver by (-)-hydroxycitrate." *Archives of Biochemistry and Biophysics* 150 (1972): 183–90.

Sullivan, A. C., J. Triscari, J. G. Hamilton, et al. "Effect of (-)-hydroxycitrate upon the Accumulation of Lipid in the Rat. I. Lipogenesis." *Lipids* 9 (1974): 121–28.

Tan, Sharon. "The Bra Connection to Breast Cancer." Frost & Sullivan, August 2002. *www.frost.com*

Theriault, A., J. T. Chao, Q. Wang, et al. "Tocotrienol: A Review of Its Therapeutic Potential." *Clinical Biochemistry* 32 (1999): 309–19 [review].

Thiel, F. J. "Natural Vitamins May Be Superior to Synthetic Ones." *Medical Hypotheses* 55, no. 6 (December 2000): 461–69.

Valenzuela, A., and A. Garrido. "Biochemical Bases of the Pharmacological Action of the Flavonoid Silymarin and of Its Structural Isomer Silibinin." *Biological Research* 27 (1994): 105–12.

"Vegetables without Vitamins." *Life Extension Magazine*, March 2001, p. 28.

Wagner, H., H. Nörr, and H. Winterhoff. "Plant Adaptogens." *Phytomedicine* 1 (1994): 63–76 [review].

Walaszek, Z., et al. "Dietary Glucarate-mediated Reduction of Sensitivity of Murine Strains to Chemical Carcinogenesis." *Cancer Letters* 33, no. 1 (October 1986): 25–32.

Wang, M., E. Fox, B. Stoecker, et al. "Serum Cholesterol of Adults Supplemented with Brewer's Yeast or Chromium Chloride." *Nutrition Research* 9 (1989): 989–98.

Wasserman, M., et al. "Organochlorine Compounds in Neoplastic and Adjacent Apparently Normal Breast Tissue." *Bulletin of Environmental Contaminants and Toxicology* 15 (1976): 478–84.

Weber, C., T. S. Jakobsen, S. A. Mortensen, et al. "Antioxidative Effect of Dietary Coenzyme Q10 in Human Blood Plasma." *International Journal for Vitamin and Nutrition Research* 64 (1994): 311–15.

West, D. B., et al. "Effects of Conjugated Linoleic Acid on Body Fat and Energy Metabolism in the Mouse." *American Journal of Physiology* 275, no. 3, part 2 (September 1998): R667–72.

Westin, J., and E. Richter. "Israeli Breast Cancer Anomaly." *Annals of the New York Academy of Sciences* 609 (1990): 269–79.

Whitaker, Julian, M.D. *Health and Healing*. Potamac, Md.: Phillips Publishing, 2002.

Wilkinson, I. B., I. L. Megson, H. MacCallum, et al. "Oral Vitamin C Reduces Arterial Stiffness and Platelet Aggregation in Humans." *Journal of Cardiovascular Pharmacology* 34 (1999): 690–93.

Wilkinson, S. C., K. H. Goulding, P. K. Robinson. "Mercury Removal by Immobilized Algae in Batch Culture Systems." *Journal of Applied Phycology* 2 (1990): 223–30.

Willett, W. C. "Is Dietary Fat a Major Determinant of Body Fat?" *American Journal of Clinical Nutrition* 67 (1998): 556–62.

Yim, C. Y., J. B. Hibbs Jr, J. R. McGregor, et al. "Use of N-acetyl Cysteine to Increase Intracellular Glutathione during the Induction of Antitumor Responses by IL-2." *Journal of Immunology* 152 (1994): 5796–805.

Yuneva, M. O., E. R. Bulygina, S. C. Gallant, et al. "Effect of Carnosine on Age-induced Changes in Senescence-accelerated Mice." *Journal of Anti-Aging Medicine* 2, no. 4 (1999): 337–42.

Zhu, Z. R., J. A. S. Mannisto, P. Pietinene, et al. "Fatty Acid Composition of Breast Adipose Tissue in Breast Cancer Patients and Patients with Benign Breast Disease." *Nutrition and Cancer* 24 (1995): 151–60.

Zi, X., D. K. Feyes, and R. Agarwal. "Anticarcinogenic Effect of a Flavonoid Antioxidant, Silymarin, in Human Breast Cancer Cells MDA-MB 468: Induction of G1 Arrest through an Increase in Cip1/p21 Concomitant with a Decrease in Kinase Activity of Cyclin-dependent Kinases and Associated Cyclins." *Clinical Cancer Research* 4, no. 4 (April 1998): 1055–64.

Ziboh, V. A., C. C. Miller, and Y. Cho. "Metabolism of Polyunsaturated Fatty Acids by Skin Epidermal Enzymes: Generation of Anti-inflammatory and Antiproliferative Metabolites. " *American Journal of Clinical Nutrition* 71, supplement 1 (2000): 361S–66S [review].

Zurier, R. B., et al. "Gamma-Linolenic Acid Treatment of Rheumatoid Arthritis: A Randomized, Placebo-controlled Trial." *Arthritis and Rheumatism* 39 (1996): 1808–17.

Chapter 9

Erasmus, Udo. *Fats That Heal, Fats That Kill.* Burnaby, B.C., Canada: Alive Books, 1986, 1993, pp. 58–59.

Frost, Phillip, M.D., and Steven Horwitz, M.D. *Principles of Cosmetics for the Dermatologist.* St. Louis, Mo.: The C. V. Mosby Company, 1982.

Kligman, A. M., and O. H. Mills. "Acne Cosmetica." *Archives of Dermatology* 106 (1972): 843–50.

Lewis, Carol. "Sunning for Science: The Effects of Common Substances on Sun-exposed Skin." *FDA Consumer* magazine, November–December 2002. *www.fda.gov/fdac/602_toc.html*

Morris, Robert, et al. "Chlorination, Chlorination By-products, and Cancer: A Meta-analysis." *American Journal of Public Health* 82, no. 7 (July 1992): 955–63.

Poole, K. "Mechanisms of Bacterial Biocide and Antibiotic Resistance." *Journal of Applied Microbiology* 92, supplement (2002): 55S–64S.

Prottey, C. "The Molecular Basis of Skin Irritation." Unilever Research Laboratory. *Cosmetic Science*, 1978.

Roeding, J., and M. Ghyczy. "Control of Skin Humidity with Liposomes: Stabilization of Skin Care Oils and Lipophillic Active Substances with Liposomes." *Seifen-Öle-Fette-Wachse (SÖFW)* 10 (1991): 378.

Schweizer, Herbert P. "Triclosan: A Widely Used Biocide and Its Link to Antibiotics." *FEMS [Federation of European Microbiological Studies] Microbiology Letters* 202, no. 1 (7 August 2001): 1–7.

Vance, Judi. *Beauty to Die For*. San Jose, Calif.: To Excel, 1999, p. 19.

Yow, Elizabeth. "Acid Washed Face: Are AHAs and Glycolics Damaging Your Skin?" *Fashion Wire Daily*, 17 November 1999. *www.fashionwiredaily.com*

Chapter 10

Berkson, D. Lindsey. *Hormone Deception*. Lincolnwood, Ill.: Contemporary Books, 2000.

Blout, B., et al. "Levels of Seven Urinary Phthalate Metabolites in a Human Reference Population." *Environmental Health Perspectives* 108 (2000): 972–82.

Bradbard, Laura. "On the Teen Scene: Cosmetics and Reality." *FDA Consumer*, November 1993, Publication No. (FDA) 94-5015.

The Cancer Prevention Coalition Web site: *www.preventcancer.com*

"Chemicals in the Environment: Toluene." Office of Pollution Prevention and Toxics, U.S. Environmental Protection Agency, August 1994. *www.epa.gov/chemfact/f_toluen.txt*

Colon, I., et al. "Identification of Phthalate Esters in the Serum of Young Puerto Rican Girls with Premature Breast Development." *Environmental Health Perspectives* 108 (2000): 895–900.

"Cosmetic Product-Related Regulatory Requirements and Health Hazard Issue." In *Cosmetic Handbook*. U.S. Food and Drug Administration Center for Food

Safety and Applied Nutrition FDA/Industry Activities Staff Booklet, 1992. *www.cfsan.fda.gov/~dms/cos-hdb3.html*

De Fazio, Angel. "How Environmentally Aware Are You?" *Holistic Times* 6, no. 3 (1999).

Epstein, Samuel, M.D., and Amy Marsh. "Perfume: Cupid's Arrow or Poison Dart?" Joint press release issued by the Cancer Prevention Coalition and the Environmental Health Network, 7 February 2002.

Epstein, Samuel S., and David R. Obey. *The Politics of Cancer Revisited*. Hankins, N.Y.: East Ridge Press, 1998.

Erickson, Kim. *Drop Dead Gorgeous*. New York: McGraw-Hill, Contemporary Books, 2002, p. 120.

Gago-Dominguez, M., J. E. Castelao, J. M. Yuan, M. C. Yu, and R. K. Ross. "Use of Permanent Hair Dyes and Bladder-cancer Risk." *International Journal of Cancer* 91, no. 4 (15 February 2001): 575–79.

Guidotti, Sylvana, William E. Wright, John Peters, M.D., et al. "Multiple Myeloma in Cosmetologists." *American Journal of Industrial Medicine* 3, no. 2 (September 1982): 169–71.

Harte, John, Cheryl Holdren, Richard Schneider, and Christine Shirley. *Toxics A to Z: A Guide to Everyday Pollution Hazards*. Berkeley and Los Angeles: University of California Press, 1991.

"Hypoallergenic Cosmetics." FDA Office of Cosmetics and Colors Fact Sheet. U.S. Food and Drug Administration. 19 December 1994, revised 18 October 2000. *www.cfsan.fda.gov/~dms/cos-224.html*

Kirkland, D. J., M.D., et al. "Hair Dye Genotoxicity." *American Heart Journal* 98, no. 6 (December 1979): 814.

Kligman, A. M., and O. Mills. "Acne Cosmetica." *Archives of Dermatology* 106 (1972): 843–50.

National Research Council. *Toxicity Testing: Strategies to Determine Needs and Priorities*. Washington, D.C.: National Academy Press, 1984.

Paustenbach, D. J. "The U.S. EPA Science Advisory Board Evaluation (2001) of the EPA Dioxin Reassessment." *Regulatory Toxicology and Pharmacology* 36, no. 2 (October 2002): 211–19.

"Public Health Statement for Toluene." U.S. Department of Health and Human Services Agency for Toxic Substances and Disease Registry. May 1994. *www.atsdr.cdc.gov/toxprofiles/phs56.html*

"Report on the Consensus Workshop on Formaldehyde." *Environmental Health Perspectives* 58 (December 1984): 323–81.

Rogers, J. M., and M. S. Denison. "Analysis of the Antiestrogenic Activity of 2,3,7,8-tetrachlorodibenzo-p-dioxin in Human Ovarian Carcinoma BG-1 Cells." *Molecular Pharmacology* 61, no. 6 (June 2002): 1393–403.

Routledge, E. J., J. Parker, J. Odum, J. Ashby, and J. P. Sumpter. "Some Alkyl Hydroxy Benzoate Preservatives (Parabens) Are Estrogenic." *Toxicology and Applied Pharmacology* 153, no. 1 (November 1998): 12–19.

Schafer, T., E. Bohler, S. Ruhdorfer, L. Weigl, D. Wessner, B. Filipiak, H. E. Wichmann, and J. Ring. "Epidemiology of Contact Allergy in Adults." *Allergy* 56, no. 12 (December 2001): 1192–96.

Scheinman, P. L. "Prevalence of Fragrance Allergy." *Dermatology* 205, no. 1 (2002): 98–102.

Schlumpf, Margaret, Beata Cotton, Marianne Conscience, Vreni Haller, Beate Steinmann, and Walter Lichtensteiger. "In Vitro and In Vivo Estrogenicity of UV Screens." *Environmental Health Perspectives* 109 (March 2001): 239–44.

Smeh, Nicholas J. *Health Risks in Today's Cosmetics.* Garrisonville, Va.: Alliance Publishing Company, 1994, p. 1.

Steinmann, David, and Samuel Epstein. *The Safe Shopper's Bible.* New York: Macmillan, 1995.

Thun, Michael J., Sean F. Alterkruse, Mohan M. Namboodiri, Eugenia E. Calle, Dena G. Meyers, and Clark W. Heath Jr. "Hair Dye Use and Risk of Fatal Cancers in U.S. Women." *Journal of the National Cancer Institute* 86 (1994): 210–15.

U.S. Department of Health and Human Services. *Cosmetics Handbook.* U.S. Food and Drug Administration Center for Food Safety and Applied Nutrition FDA/Industry Activities Staff Booklet. Washington, D.C.: U.S. Government Printing Office, 1992.

Winter, Ruth. *A Consumer's Dictionary of Cosmetic Ingredients.* New York: Crown, 1989, p. 9.

Yu, M. C., P. L. Skipper, S. R. Tannenbaum, K. K. Chan, and R. K. Ross. "Arylamine Exposures and Bladder Cancer Risk." *Mutation Research* 506–7 (30 September 2002): 21–28 [review].

Chapter 11

Abels, D. J., T. Rose, and J. E. Bearman. "Treatment of Psoriasis at a Dead Sea Dermatology Clinic." *International Journal of Dermatology* 34, no. 2 (February 1995): 134–37.

Aertgeerts, P., et al. "Comparative Testing of Kamillosan Cream and Steroidal (0.25% Hydrocortisone, 0.75% Fluocortin Butyl Ester) and Non-steroidal (5% Bufexamac) Dermatologic Agents in Maintenance Therapy of Eczematous Diseases" (in German). *Zeitschrift für Hautkrankheiten* 60, no. 3 (1985): 270–77.

Aesoph, Lauri. *Your Natural Health Makeover.* Upper Saddle River, N.J.: Prentice Hall, 1998.

Allison, J. R. "The Relation of Hydrochloric Acid and Vitamin B Complex Deficiency in Certain Skin Diseases." *Southern Medical Journal* 38 (1945): 235–41.

Almas, K. "Antimicrobial Effects of Extracts of Azadirachta Indica (Neem) and Salvadora Persica (Arak) Chewing Sticks." *Indian Journal of Dental Research* 10 (January–March 1999): 23–26.

Angermeier, M. C. "Treatment of Facial Vascular Lesions with Intense Pulsed Light." *Journal of Cutaneous Laser Therapy* 1, no. 2 (April 1999): 95–100.

"Azelaic Acid—A New Topical Treatment for Acne." *Drug and Therapy Bulletin* 31 (1993): 50–52.

Berbis, P., S. Hesse, and Y. Privat. "Essential Fatty Acids and the Skin." *Allergie et Immunologie* (Paris) 22, no. 6 (June 1990): 225–31.

Bernstein, J. E., L. C. Parish, M. Rapaport, M. M. Rosenbaum, and H. H. Roenigk Jr. "Effects of Topically Applied Capsaicin on Moderate and Severe Psoriasis Vulgaris." *Journal of the American Academy of Dermatology* 15, no. 3 (September 1986): 504–7.

Bierhaus, A., et al. "Advanced Glycation End Product-induced Activation of NF-kappaB Is Suppressed by Alpha-lipoic Acid in Cultured Endothelial Cells." *Diabetes* 46, no. 9 (September 1997): 1481–90.

Blumenthal, Mark, Alicia Goldberg, and Josef Brinckmann. *Herbal Medicine: Expanded Commission E Monographs.* Newton, Mass.: Integrative Medicine Communications, 2000.

Boelsma, E., H. F. Hendriks, and L. Roza. "Nutritional Skin Care: Health Effects of Micronutrients and Fatty Acids." *American Journal of Clinical Nutrition* 73, no. 5 (May 2001): 853–64.

Brownstein, Arlen, M.S., N.D., and Donna Schoemaker, C.N. *Rosacea: Your Self-Help Guide*. Oakland, Calif.: Harbinger Publications, 2001.

Chithra, P., et al. "Influence of Aloe Vera on Collagen Characteristics in Healing Dermal Wounds in Rats." *Molecular and Cellular Biochemistry* 181, nos. 1–2 (April 1998): 71–76.

Cordain, L., S. Lindeberg, M. Hurtado, K. Hill, S. B. Eaton, and J. Brand-Miller. "Acne Vulgaris: A Disease of Western Civilization." *Archives of Dermatology* 138, no. 12 (December 2002): 1584–90.

Diehm, C., H. J. Trampisch, S. Lange, and C. Schmidt. "Comparison of Leg Compression Stocking and Oral Horse-chestnut Seed Extract Therapy in Patients with Chronic Venous Insufficiency." *Lancet* 347, no. 8997 (3 February 1996): 292–94.

Diehm C., D. Vollbrecht, K. Amendt, and H. U. Comberg. "Medical Edema Protection—Clinical Benefit in Patients with Chronic Deep Vein Incompetence: A Placebo-controlled Double-blind Study." *Vasa* 21, no. 2 (1992): 188–92.

Dreno, B., D. Moyse, M. Alirezai, P. Amblard, N. Auffret, C. Beylot, I. Bodokh, M. Chivot, F. Daniel, P. Humbert, J. Meynadier, and F. Poli. "Multicenter Randomized Comparative Double-blind Controlled Clinical Trial of the Safety and Efficacy of Zinc Gluconate versus Minocycline Hydrochloride in the Treatment of Inflammatory Acne Vulgaris." *Dermatology* 203, no. 2 (2001): 135–40.

Ellis, C. N., et al. "A Double-blind Evaluation of Topical Capsaicin in Pruritic Psoriasis." *Journal of the American Academy of Dermatology* 29, no. 3 (September 1993): 438–42.

Evans, F. Q. "The Rational Use of Glycyrrhetinic Acid in Dermatology." *British Journal of Clinical Practice* 12 (1958): 269–79.

Fitton, A., and K. L. Goa. "Azelaic Acid: A Review of Its Pharmacological Properties and Therapeutic Efficacy in Acne and Hyperpigmentary Skin Disorders." *Drugs* 41 (1991): 780–98.

Fitzpatrick, R. E., and E. F. Rostan. "Double-blind, Half-face Study Comparing Topical Vitamin C and Vehicle for Rejuvenation of Photodamage." *Dermatologic Surgery* 28, no. 3 (March 2002): 231–36.

Fluhr, J. W., J. Kao, M. Jain, S. K. Ahn, K. R. Feingold, and P. M. Elias. "Generation of Free Fatty Acids from Phospholipids Regulates Stratum Corneum Acidification and Integrity." *Journal of Investigative Dermatology* 117, no. 1 (July 2001): 44–51.

Frost, Phillip, M.D., and Steven N. Horwitz. *Principles of Cosmetics for the Dermatologist*. St. Louis, Mo.: The C. V. Mosby Company, 1982.

Fu, M. X., J. R. Requena, A. J. Jenkins, T. J. Lyons, J. W. Baynes, and S. R.Thorpe. "The Advanced Glycation End-product, Ne-(carboxymethyl)lysine, Is a Product of Both Lipid Peroxidation and Glycoxidation Reactions." *Journal of Biological Chemistry* 271 (1996): 9982–86.

Gieler, U., A. von der Weth, and M. Heger. "Mahonia Aquifolium—a New Type of Topical Treatment for Psoriasis." *Journal of Dermatological Treatment* 6, no. 1 (March 1995): 31–34.

Gollnick, H. P., and A. Krautheim. "Topical Treatment in Acne: Durrent Status and Future Aspects." *Dermatology* 206, no. 1 (2003): 29–36.

Hahn, G. S. "Strontium Is a Potent and Selective Inhibitor of Sensory Irritation." *Dermatologic Surgery* 25, no. 9 (September 1999): 689–94.

Horrobin, D. F. "The Importance of Gamma-linolenic Acid and Prostaglandin E1 in Human Nutrition and Medicine." *Journal of Holistic Medicine* 3 (1981): 118–39.

Katiyar, S. K., B. M. Bergamo, P. K. Vyalil, and C. A. Elmets. "Green Tea Polyphenols: DNA Photodamage and Photoimmunology." *Journal of Photochemistry and Photobiology* 65, nos. 2–3 (31 December 2001): 109–14.

Kumagai, A., M. Nanaboshi, Y. Asanuma, et al. "Effects of Glycyrrhizin on Thymolytic and Immunosuppressive Action of Cortisone." *Endocrinologia Japonica* 14 (1967): 39–42.

Kunt, T., et al. "Alpha-lipoic Acid Reduces Expression of Vascular Cell Adhesion Molecule-1 and Endothelial Adhesion of Human Monocytes after Stimulation with Advanced Glycation End Products." *Clinical Science* (London) 96, no. 1 (January 1999): 75–82.

Lautenschlager, H., J. Roeding, and M. Ghyczy. "The Use of Liposomes from Soybean Phospholipids in Cosmetics." *Seifen-Öle-Fette-Wachse (SÖFW)* 14, no. 88: 531–34.

Letawe, C., M. Boone, and G. E. Pierard. "Digital Image Analysis of the Effect of Topically Applied Linoleic Acid on Acne Microcomedones." *Clinical Experimental Dermatology* 23, no. 2 (March 1998): 56–58.

Liao, S. "Androgen Action: Molecular Mechanism and Medical Application." *Journal of the Formosan Medical Association* 93, no. 9 (September 1994): 741–51.

Lingelbach, L. B., A. E. Mitchell, R. B. Rucker, and R. B. McDonald. "Accumulation of Advanced Glycation Endproducts in Aging Male Fischer 344 Rats During

Long-term Feeding of Various Dietary Carbohydrates." *Journal of Nutrition* 130, no. 5 (May 2000): 1247–55.

Maurice, P. D. L., B. R. Allen, A. S. J. Barkley, et al. "The Effects of Dietary Supplementation with Fish Oil in Patients with Psoriasis." *British Journal of Dermatology* 1117 (1987): 599–606.

McFarland, G. A., and R. Holliday. "Retardation of the Senescence of Cultured Human Diploid Fibroblasts by Carnosine." *Experimental Cell Research* 212, no. 2 (1994): 167–75.

Morrissey, Stephen. "Incurable No Longer: An Extract from the Oregon Grape Eliminates Psoriasis Suffering." *Health Sciences Member Alert*, December 1999, p. 5.

Murray, Michael T., N.D. *Natural Alternatives to Over-the-Counter and Prescription Drugs.* New York: William Morrow, 1994.

Nguyen, Q. H., and T. P. Bui. "Azelaic Acid: Pharmacokinetic and Pharmacodynamic Properties and Its Therapeutic Role in Hyperpigmentary Disorders and Acne." *International Journal of Dermatology* 34 (1995): 75–84.

Perricone, Nicholas, M.D. *The Perricone Prescription.* New York: HarperCollins: 2002.

Putzier, E. "Dermatomycoses and an Antifungal Diet." *Wiener Medizinische Wochenschrift* 139, nos. 15–16 (31 August 1989): 379–80.

Reynolds, T., et al. "Aloe Vera Leaf Gel: A Review Update." *Journal of Ethnopharmacology* 68, nos. 1–3 (December 1999): 3–37.

Roan, S. "Worship Your Skin." *Argus Leader*, 30 July 1996.

Smeh, Nicholas J. *Health Risks in Today's Cosmetics.* Garrisonville, Va.: Alliance Publishing Company, 1994, p. 33.

Traber, M. G., et al. "Diet Derived Topically Applied Tocotrienols Accumulate in Skin and Protect the Tissue against UV Light-induced Oxidative Stress." *Asia Pacific Journal of Clinical Nutrition* 6 (1997): 63–67.

Trowell, H., D. Burkitt, and K. Heaton. *Dietary Fiber, Fiber-Depleted Foods and Disease.* London: Academic Press, 1985.

Walker, M. "Astonishing Healing of Psoriasis Using the Euro-import." *Townsend Letter*, January 1997, pp. 58–64.

Warner, R. R., J. R. Schwartz, Y. Boissy, and T. L. Dawson Jr. "Dandruff Has an Altered Stratum Corneum Ultrastructure That Is Improved with Zinc Pyrithione Shampoo." *Journal of the American Academy of Dermatology* 45, no. 6 (December 2001): 897–903.

Ziboh, V. A. "Prostaglandins, Leukotrienes, and Hydroxy Fatty Acids in Epidermis." *Seminars in Dermatology* 11, no. 2 (June 1992): 114–20.

Ziboh, V. A., and C. C. Miller. "Essential Fatty Acids and Polyunsaturated Fatty Acids: Significance in Cutaneous Biology." *Annual Review of Nutrition* 10 (1990): 433–50.

Chapter 12

Abou-Donia, M. "Use Caution When Using DEET." Duke Health Note, July 2002. *www.dukehealth.org/news/healthtip_julyo2.asp*

Allen, P. "Tea Tree Oil: The Science Behind the Antimicrobial Hype." *Journal of Antimicrobial Chemotherapy* 48 (2001): 450.

Amin, A. H., et al. "Berberine Sulfate: Antimicrobial Activity, Bioassay, and Mode of Action." *Canadian Journal of Microbiology* 15 (1969): 1067–76.

Aridogan, B. C., H. Baydar, S. Kaya, M. Demirci, D. Ozbasar, and E. Mumcu. "Antimicrobial Activity and Chemical Composition of Some Essential Oils." *Archives of Pharmacal Research* 25, no. 6 (December 2002): 860–64.

Balch, James F., M.D., and Phyllis A. Balch, C.N.C. *Prescription for Nutritional Healing*, 3rd ed. New York: Avery Penguin Putnam, 2000.

Bauer, V. R., K. Jurcic, J. Puhlmann, et al. "Immunologic In Vivo and In Vitro Studies on Echinacea Extracts." *Arzneimittelforschung* 38, no. 2 (February 1988): 276–81.

Bronner, C., and Y. Landry. "Kinetics of the Inhibitory Effect of Flavonoids on Histamine Secretion from Mast Cells." *Agents Actions* 16 (1985): 147–51.

Buck, D. S., D. M. Nidorf, and J. G. Addino. "Comparison of Two Topical Preparations for the Treatment of Onychomycosis: Melaleuca Alternifolia (Tea Tree) Oil and Clotrimazole." *Journal of Family Practice* 38, no. 6 (June 1994): 601–5.

Caelli, M., J. Porteous, C. F. Carson, R. Heller, and T. V. Riley. "Tea Tree Oil as an Alternative Topical Decolonization Agent for Methicillin-resistant Staphylococcus Aureus." *Journal of Hospital Infection* 46, no. 3 (November 2000): 236–37.

Carson, C. F., B. J. Mee, and T. V. Riley. "Mechanism of Action of Melaleuca Alternifolia (Tea Tree) Oil on Staphylococcus Aureus Determined by Time-kill, Lysis, Leakage, and Salt Tolerance Assays and Electron Microscopy." *Antimicrobial Agents and Chemotherapy* 46, no. 6 (June 2002): 1914–20.

Cramer, Daniel W., et al. "Ovarian Cancer and Talc: A Case-Control Study." *Cancer* 50 (15 July 1982): 372–76.

Dry, J., and D. Vincent. "Effect of a Fish Oil Diet on Asthma: Results of a One-year Double-blind Study." *International Archives of Allergy and Applied Immunology* 95, nos. 2–3 (1991): 156–57.

Hay, I. C., M. Jamieson, and A. D. Ormerod. "Randomized Trial of Aromatherapy: Successful Treatment for Alopecia Areata." *Archives of Dermatology* 134, no. 11 (November 1998): 1349–52.

Heggers, J. P., J. Cottingham, J. Gusman, L. Reagor, L. McCoy, E. Carino, R. Cox, J. G. Zhao, and L. Reagor. "The Effectiveness of Processed Grapefruit-seed Extract as an Antibacterial Agent: II. Mechanism of Action and In Vitro Toxicity." *Journal of Alternative and Complementary Medicine* 8, no. 3 (June 2002): 333–40.

Hirt, M., S. Nobel, and E. Barron. "Zinc Nasal Gel for the Treatment of Common Cold Symptoms: A Double-blind, Placebo-Controlled Trial." *Ear, Nose, and Throat Journal* 79, no. 10 (October 2000): 778–80, 782.

Ionescu, G., R. Kiehl, F. Wichmann-Kunz, et al. "Oral Citrus Seed Extract in Atopic Eczema: In Vitro and In Vivo Studies on Intestinal Microflora." *Journal of Orthomolecular Medicine* 5 (1990): 155–58.

Lassus, A., et al. "A Comparative Study of a New Food Supplement, Viviscal, with Fish Extract for the Treatment of Hereditary Androgenic Alopecia in Young Males." *The Journal of International Medical Research* 20 (1992): 445–53.

Lassus, A., J. Santalahti, and M. Sellmann. "Treatment of Hereditary Androgenic Alopecia in Middle-aged Males by Combined Oral and Topical Administration of Special Marine Extract-Compound (Viviscal)." *Les Nouvelles Dermatologiques* 13 (1994): 254–55.

Luettig, B., et al. "Macrophage Activation by the Polysaccharide Arabinogalactan Isolated from Plant Cell Cultures of Echinacea Purpurea." *Journal of the American Cancer Institute* 81, no. 9 (1989): 669–75.

Manohar, V., C. Ingram, J. Gray, N. A. Talpur, B. W. Echard, D. Bagchi, and H. G. Preuss. "Antifungal Activities of Origanum Oil against Candida Albicans." *Molecular and Cellular Biochemistry* 228, nos. 1–2 (December 2001): 111–17.

Mercola, Joseph M., D.O. "Oregano, Other Essential Oils Destroy Strep Pneumonia Cells." *Townsend Letter*, August/September 1998.

Mittman, P. "Randomized, Double-blind Study of Freeze-dried Urtica Dioica in the Treatment of Allergic Rhinitis." *Planta Medica* 56 (1990): 44–47.

National Nutritional Foods Association Web site: *www.nnfa.org*

Ooshima, T., T. Minami, W. Aono, et al. "Reduction of Dental Plaque Deposition in Humans by Oolong Tea Extract." *Caries Research* 28 (1994): 146–49.

Oyedele, A. O., A. A. Gbolade, M. B. Sosan, F. B. Adewoyin, O. L. Soyelu, and O. O. Orafidya. "Formulation of an Effective Mosquito-repellant Topical Product from Lemongrass Oil." *Phytomedicine* 9, no. 3 (April 2002): 259–62.

Prager, N., K. Bickett, N. French, and G. Marcovici. "A Randomized, Double-blind, Placebo-controlled Trial to Determine the Effectiveness of Botanically Derived Inhibitors of 5-alpha-reductase in the Treatment of Androgenetic Alopecia." *Journal of Alternative and Complementary Medicine* 8, no. 2 (April 2002): 143–52.

Rabbani, G. H., et al. "Randomized Controlled Trial of Berberine Sulfate Therapy for Diarrhea Due to Enterotoxigenic Escherichia Coli and Vibrio Cholerae." *The Journal of Infectious Diseases* 155, no. 5 (1987): 979–84.

Ratner, P. H., P. M. Ehrlich, S. M. Fineman, E. O. Meltzer, and D. P. Skoner. "Use of Intranasal Cromolyn Sodium for Allergic Rhinitis." *Mayo Clinic: Proceedings* 77, no. 4 (April 2002): 350–54.

Reagor, L., J. Gusman, L. McCoy, E. Carino, and J. P. Heggers. "The Effectiveness of Processed Grapefruit-seed Extract as an Antibacterial Agent: I. An In Vitro Agar Assay." *Journal of Alternative and Complementary Medicine* 8, no. 3 (June 2002): 325–32.

Reid, G. "The Role of Cranberry and Probiotics in Intestinal and Urogenital Tract Health." *Critical Reviews in Food Science and Nutrition* 42, supplement 3 (2002): 293–300.

Roesler, J., A. Emmendorffer, C. Steinmuller, et al. "Application of Purified Polysaccharides from Cell Cultures of the Plant Echinacea purpurea to Test Subjects Mediates Activation of the Phagocyte System." *International Journal of Immunopharmacology* 13, no. 7 (1991): 931–41.

"The Safety of Sporanox Capsules and Lamisil Tablets for the Treatment of Onychomycosis." FDA Public Health Advisory, 9 May 2001. *www.fda.gov/cder/drug/advisory/sporanox-lamisil/advisory.htm*

Schlumpf, Margaret, Beata Cotton, Marianne Conscience, Vreni Haller, Beate Steinmann, and Walter Lichtensteiger. "In Vitro and In Vivo Estrogenicity of UV Screens." *Environmental Health Perspectives* 109 (March 2001): 239–44.

Thompson, K. D. "Antiviral Activity of Viracea against Acyclovir Susceptible and Acyclovir Resistant Strains of Herpes Simplex Virus." *Antiviral Research* 39, no. 1 (July 1998): 55–61.

Uhari, M., et al. "Xylitol in Preventing Acute Otitis Media." *Vaccine* 19, supplement 1 (2000): S144–47.

U.S. Food and Drug Administration, Center for Drug Evaluation and Research Approval Letter. Nasalcrom. Application No. 20-463/S-002, 27 March 2001.

Winn, D. M., W. J. Blot, J. K. McLaughlin, D. F. Austin, R. S. Greenberg, S. Preston-Martin, J. B. Schoenberg, and J. F. Fraumeni Jr. "Mouthwash Use and Oral Conditions in the Risk of Oral and Pharyngeal Cancer." *Cancer Research* 51, no. 11 (1 June 1991): 3044–47.

Xiong, H., Y. Li, M. F. Slavik, and J. Walker. "Spraying Chicken Skin with Selected Chemicals to Reduce Attached Salmonella Typhimurium." *Journal of Food Protection* 61 (1998): 272–75.

Zabner, J., et al. "The Osmolyte Xylitol Reduces the Salt Concentration of Airway Surface Liquid and May Enhance Bacterial Killing." *Proceedings of the National Academy of Sciences* (USA) 97 (10 October 2000): 11614–19.

Chapter 13

Bouic, P. J. D., P. P. van Jaarsveld, A. Clark, J. H. Lamprecht, M. Freestone, and R. W. Liebenberg. "The Effects of B-sitosterol (BSS) and B-sitosterol Glucoside (BSSG) Mixture on Selected Immune Parameters of Marathon Runners: Inhibition of Post Marathon Immune Suppression and Inflammation." *International Journal of Sports Medicine* 20 (1999): 258–62.

Brown, David. "Women Taking Another Look at Ways to Treat Menopause Problems with Hormone Therapy May Boost Other Remedies." *The Washington Post*, 29 August 2002, p. A03.

Bunevicius, Robertas, G. Kazanavicius, R. Zalinkevicius, A. J. Prange Jr. "Effects of Thyroxine as Compared with Thyroxine Plus Triiodothyronine in Patients with Hypothyroidism." *New England Journal of Medicine* 340, no. 6 (11 February 1999): 424–29.

Cherniske, Stephen. *Caffeine Blues*. New York: Warner Books, 1998.

Düker, E. M., L. Kopanski, H. Jarry, and W. Wuttke. "Effects of Extracts from Cimicifuga Racemosa on Gonadotropin Release in Menopausal Women and Ovariectomized Rats." *Planta Medica* 57 (1991): 420–24.

Ferri, J. "Under Pressure." *Tampa Tribune-Times*, 27 April 1997.

Gaby, A. R. "Treatment with Thyroid Hormone." *Journal of the American Medical Association* 262, no. 13 (6 October 1989): 1774–75.

Khatri, Parinda, James A. Blumenthal, Michael A. Babyak, W. Edward Craighead, Steve Herman, Teri Baldewicz, David J. Madden, Murali Doraiswamy, Robert Waugh, and K. Ranga Krishnan. "Effects of Exercise Training on Cognitive Functioning Among Depressed Older Men and Women." *Journal of Aging and Physical Activity* 9, no. 1 (2001): 43.

Kolata, Gina. "Citing Risks, U.S. Will Halt Study of Drugs for Hormones." *The New York Times*, 9 June 2002.

Lark, Susan M. "Research Corner: Coffee Increases Estrogen Levels." *The Lark Letter* 9, no. 3 (March 2000) (Phillips Health, LLC, Potomac, Maryland).

Lark, Susan M. "Research on HRT, Soy, and Vitamin C." *The Lark Letter* 9, no. 4 (April 2000).

Lark, Susan M. "Undoing Estrogen Dominence." *The Lark Letter* 9, no. 3 (March 2000).

Lazarou, J., B. H. Pomeranz, and P. N. Corey. "Incidence of Adverse Drug Reactions in Hospitalized Patients: A Meta-analysis of Prospective Studies." *Journal of the American Medical Association* 279, no. 15 (15 April 1998): 1200–1205.

Lehmann-Willenbrock, E., and H.-H. Riedel. "Clinical and Endocrinologic Examination Concerning Therapy of Climacteric Symptoms Following Hysterectomy with Remaining Ovaries." *Zentralblatt Gynäkologie* 110 (1988): 611–18.

Lucero, J., B. L. Harlow, R. L. Barbieri, P. Sluss, and D. W. Cramer. "Early Follicular Phase Hormone Levels in Relation to Patterns of Alcohol, Tobacco, and Coffee Use." *Fertility and Sterility* 76, no. 4 (October 2001): 723–29.

Ray, Paul H., and Sherry Ruth Anderson. *The Cultural Creatives: How Fifty Million People Are Changing the World.* New York: Harmony Books, 2000.

Rosignol, Annette MacKay. "Caffeine-containing Beverages and Premenstrual Syndrome in Young Women." *American Journal of Public Health* 75 (1985): 1335–37.

Stoll, W. "Phytopharmacon Influences Atrophic Vaginal Epithelium: Double Blind Study—*Cimicifuga* vs. Estrogenic Substances." *Therapeuticum* 1 (1987): 23–31.

Warnecke, G. "Influencing Menopausal Symptoms with a Phytotherapeutic Agent: Successful Therapy with Cimicifuga Mono-extract." *Medizinische Welt* 36 (1985): 871–74.

index

Beyond Words Publishing, Inc.

OUR CORPORATE MISSION
Inspire to Integrity

OUR DECLARED VALUES
We give to all of life as life has given us.
We honor all relationships.
Trust and stewardship are integral to fulfilling dreams.
Collaboration is essential to create miracles.
Creativity and aesthetics nourish the soul.
Unlimited thinking is fundamental.
Living your passion is vital.
Joy and humor open our hearts to growth.
It is important to remind ourselves of love.

To order or to request a catalog, contact

Beyond Words Publishing, Inc.
20827 N.W. Cornell Road, Suite 500
Hillsboro, OR 97124-9808
503-531-8700

You can also visit our Web site at *www.beyondword.com*
or e-mail us at *info@beyondword.com*.